NO HOUSE CALLS

IRREVERENT NOTES ON THE PRACTICE OF MEDICINE

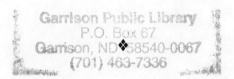
BY PETER GOTT, M.D.

POSEIDON PRESS, NEW YORK

DESIGNED BY BARBARA MARKS

MANUFACTURED IN THE UNITED STATES OF AMERICA

1 3 5 7 9 10 8 6 4 2

LIBRARY OF CONGRESS CATALOGING IN PUBLICATION DATA
GOTT, PETER, DATE
  NO HOUSE CALLS.

  1. MEDICINE—UNITED STATES. 2. PHYSICIANS—UNITED
STATES. 3. MEDICINE—UNITED STATES—ANECDOTES, FA-
CETIAE, SATIRE, ETC. 4. PHYSICIANS—UNITED STATES—
ANECDOTES, FACETIAE, SATIRE, ETC. I. TITLE.
R151.G6 1986   610'.92'2   86-16963
ISBN: 0-671-60433-3

ACKNOWLEDGMENTS

My sincere thanks go to David Hendin, senior vice-president and editorial director of United Media. He took me on as a project because he believed in what I had to say, and he taught me that consumer advocacy is a concept that embodies the highest ideals of the medical profession. His confidence, guidance and direction have helped me enormously.

I am grateful to Elaine Pfefferblit, my editor, for her vision and commitment to organizing the thoughts and perspectives of this book into a coherent entity. My gratitude also goes to all those at Simon and Schuster who helped create, design and promote the book.

I appreciate the encouragement and stick-to-itiveness of several newspaper editors and publishers, including Stewart Hoskins, Bob Estabrook and Lawrence K. Miller.

I want to thank Dr. Lewis Thomas for unknowingly kindling my interest in medical writing because of his unique and readable style. His "Notes of a Biology Watcher" in the *New England Journal of Medicine* first taught me that writing by a doctor could be fun to read.

I also thank my many medical colleagues without whom this book would not have been possible. They showed me the best and the worst in our profession. They have always provided stimulating material and, I predict, will continue to do so.

I am grateful to Helen Canevari, my secretary for many years, for the extra time she took out of many busy days to type another column, week after week. I am also grateful to Ann Miller for preparing the manuscript in short order, when the crunch was on.

I owe my greatest debt and acknowledgment to my patients—old and young, poor or wealthy, trustful or suspicious, difficult or easy, dangerously ill or simply troubled by minor ailments. No matter. They educated me and taught me what it means to be a patient caught up in a medical system that seems calculated to remove modesty, ignore independence and require that the ill often subjugate their own rights to those of the system. To the patients who have been loyal and have given me their wholehearted support and encouragement, I am most grateful.

Finally, I want to thank the many readers of my newspaper column, who have taken the time and trouble to write me their questions, suggestions, concerns and complaints. I include them in my "practice" and am grateful to them for taking me into their lives and homes—and sharing with me their frustrations and successes. It is the public's pulse, transmitted to me by comments and in letters, that lets me know I am doing a good job and providing a service—in the form of literary house calls.

TO JUDITH, MY WIFE,
WHO HAS PUT UP WITH MORE THAN
I'LL EVER KNOW

CONTENTS

FOREWORD

Medical practice is changing. Some of these changes are patient-oriented and some are not. In a few years, much of the scientific material in this book will be outdated. New diagnostic tools, new cures and new ways of looking at disease will alter doctors' practices as well as patients' experiences with the medical profession. Nonetheless, I believe that the supporting beams of this book—having to do with the basic ways we view health, disease and each other—will remain valid well into the next century. Humanism and caring must always be medical priorities. Patients need not be intimidated by science and the health profession. The process of questioning authority and demanding answers will, in the long run, strengthen rather than weaken both the patient's relation to his or her doctor and the doctor's own relation to his career and profession. Pomposity, arrogance and greed have plagued the healing arts for hundreds of years. However, modern medicine—with all its wonders—does not excuse the continuation of these character flaws in doctors. If we physicians are going to survive as a profession, we must address these issues and not assume that they characterize only a small minority of healers. Hubris, elitism and exploitation have no place in treating the sick. Our strength, as a profession, has always been that we have been willing to make patients' needs preeminent. Most of today's doctors continue this fine tradition. If the tradition is to continue—

and I believe that it must—the public has to demand it and, at the same time, recognize that doctors, being human, are no better or no worse than the patients they serve.

INTRODUCTION

I belong to a club. Although it is not particularly exclusive, it is expensive to join.

In the early 1960s, when I attended medical school, I was totally dependent on my family for tuition, room, food, books and other fundamental expenses. This commitment cost several thousand dollars a year. (For today's medical students, it is much more.) However, my father gladly bore this "initiation fee," and I am grateful to him for the sacrifice he and my mother made at the time. It was worth it. No one ever said that joining the Medical Club would be cheap; but the M.D. degree carries so many perquisites that, in my wildest dreams, I could never have conceived what a sound investment medical school could be. But I am getting ahead of my story.

I was an army brat. During the years before World War II, my family moved annually. My life was constantly disrupted. I learned to survive new schools, new neighborhoods, new friends—and new bullies. Although I chose to become a people-pleaser, I never had a feeling of fitting in. Only during the past few years have I come to realize how disorganized my early life was, especially after my father left for three years of active duty with General Patton's Third Army when I was seven.

After the war, he returned home and we moved to Scarsdale, New York. There, for the first time, I began to enjoy some consistency in my life. I was able to sharpen my survival techniques, the same methods that would stand me in such good stead throughout my later medical career. I became competitive and superficially independent. I learned that I would be accepted or rejected depending on my manner and appearance. Without realizing it, I was already preening myself for the medical profession.

Despite my average intellect, I performed well in high school. Gregariousness and capability were values I cultivated. I was involved in extracurricular activities, played acceptable jazz piano and became a ranked tennis player. I think I was an awful phony.

In 1953, I was accepted to Princeton University, where I enrolled in the minimum premedical curriculum. I preferred courses in psychology, sociology and literature, in distinction to the orientations of other premeds who thrived on science. In those days, high-school graduates rarely fitted the Princeton "preppy" image. Although I never felt that I fit into the high-altitude atmosphere at Princeton, the university certainly fit into my plans. I was on the freshman swim team and, later, became the music director of Princeton's nationally known close-harmony singing group, the Nassoons. As a sociology major, I graduated with what was then considered to be "a gentleman's C" average. I then took a year of graduate work in the Princeton department of psychology. Midway through that year, I was accepted at Tulane Medical School. I took the big plunge in 1958.

I was not intellectually or emotionally prepared for medical school. I frankly admit I wouldn't be prepared for it today were I required to repeat the experience. The work was far more difficult than I had imagined and, early on, required agonizing memorization of details that seemed to have no relation to healing the sick. I came close to flunking out my first year. However, I decided that since I'd made a commitment, I was going to stick to it, come hell or high water. Hell did come that summer as I retook gross anatomy in an un-air-conditioned lab during New Orleans' hottest and most humid season.

In some as yet unexplained way, my survival instinct carried me through. I adapted, I worked and I progressively improved my academic standing until, finally, I graduated in the top half of my class. Not a brilliant record but, as I was later to appreciate, it's the post-medical-school training that really counts. I estimate that 60 percent of what was taught in medical-school classrooms I never used, 30 percent was incorrect and about 10 percent was potentially valuable. We were taught the science of medicine; what we learned was how to behave like doctors. This is a fine distinction, but it is an important one. Doctor behavior, like the habits of any self-styled elite group, is learned and practiced and sharpened. As you will see in this book, it often contradicts the idealistic and humanistic convictions that drive many young men and women to undergo deprivation in their quest for an M.D. degree.

The Intern Matching Program was good to me. I was accepted at Mount Sinai Hospital in New York City. To this day, I believe that I was picked to fulfill Mount Sinai's geographic mix: I was a northern Protestant from a southern school. My year at Mount Sinai was splendid, challenging and intellectually rewarding. It opened doors for me. It was also sordid, exhausting and frustrating. For the first time, I began to perceive clearly the varied ways in which the medical profession willfully depreciates, exploits and harms patients. To use a military analogy, medical school was prolonged boot camp and basic training; internship was the first active duty in combat—and, you better believe, it was war.

Mount Sinai in the 1960s was a large teaching hospital renowned for its intellectualism. Subsequently, it added a medical school, but when I was there it was a sprawling complex of private pavilions, clinics, on-call rooms, laboratories, amphitheaters and the wards. The wards were whole floors to which middle-income and indigent patients were admitted for medical and surgical care. Interns and residents trained on the wards. We learned how to perform procedures, to diagnose disease and to treat patients who were, for all practical purposes, our property. There was a tradition on the wards: the interns were ex-

pected to establish a diagnosis and outline a plan of treatment
before they went to bed.

This policy had its drawbacks. There was rarely a problem
for patients admitted during the day: they got "worked up" and
taken care of before sunset. However, when sick people entered
the hospital at night—especially after midnight—neither they
nor the doctors-in-training could "pack it in" until the diagnosis
had been made. Often the exercise took the rest of the night.

For interns, this policy was a matter of pride; for patients,
it took the form of prolonged discomfort and exhaustion. A
3 A.M. barium enema examination, preceded and followed by
batteries of blood tests, may have been a medical challenge for
a white-coated savior, but it was a nightmare for an elderly sick
man who had the misfortune to have been brought to the hospital
at 1 A.M. for rectal bleeding.

I remember Mrs. Goldfarb, white and fragile in her hospital
bed. Her arms were masses of bruises where inexperienced
interns had honed their blood-drawing skills. The young doctors
drew the early-morning blood samples in those days, and because we were sleepy and unskilled we sometimes had to try
several times to obtain blood from patients with "bad veins."
We kept trying until we got it. Mrs. Goldfarb was a living testimonial to our lack of expertise. Yet, each morning before
breakfast, she threw out her frail blue arms for the daily ritual,
and each morning she would sigh contentedly: "God bless you
young doctors!" After about a week of this, her attitude suddenly
changed. "God damn you young doctors!" she snarled at a sweating new intern as he probed her arm for the elusive vein. A
classic case of passive aggression, we were told. Happens all
the time. I wondered. I speculated about how I would behave
if I were in her position, and I began to realize the magnitude
of the enormous trade-off: our education versus patient comfort,
us versus them. That realization has haunted me ever since. I
don't ever want to forget that first crack in the concrete foundation of elitism.

I chose to take my residency in internal medicine at St.
Luke's Hospital, on the west side of Manhattan, at the edge of

Spanish Harlem. St. Luke's is now affiliated with Columbia Presbyterian Medical Center and was merged with Roosevelt Hospital. I trained there before the merger. In those days, it was genteel, upper-crust, even elegant. There was a jovial conviviality, "vespers" (cocktails) on the roof every Friday afternoon, and an endless supply of nurses and nursing students. After the fire battle of internship, I felt in my residency that I had been sent back to division headquarters for a little R & R.

There were good times and there were bad. I learned a great deal. I learned to respect patients and to be kind to them. Some of the caring feelings I had had in my first year of medical school came back to me. That felt good. I respected the attending physicians I worked under. In my final (third) year of residency, I rotated through the pulmonary division at Bellevue Hospital and discovered that the battle between the self-interest of the training doctor and the comfort of the patient still raged. I vowed never to practice medicine in a city. I knew I needed more from my profession than a Park Avenue address and a part-time teaching position in a prestigious medical center.

After my formal training, I migrated to rural Connecticut. I have practiced here, in general medicine, for twenty years. It is a good life. I enjoy my work.

Soon after I came to this New England town, I became infected with an incurable ailment: writing. In 1967 I read that housewives, who wanted additional cleaning power, were mixing household ammonia with chlorine bleach. The chemical reaction liberated chlorine gas, which made cleaning much more of a chore than the ladies anticipated because they could not breathe. I wrote a short summary of the report and presented it to the editor of the town's weekly newspaper. He published it as a public service and asked for more. I began writing a biweekly health column called "Doctor in the House."

In the beginning, I wrote informational material: how to treat sprains, how to get rings off swollen fingers, what to do about sore throats and diarrhea. As the years passed and I gained perspective, I began to address more general issues. I became increasingly concerned about doctors' attitudes, the inconsistencies in the health-care profession, the methods by which physicians keep patients "in their places," the increasing "us" (the medical guild) versus "them" (the public) mentality.

Rather than point accusing fingers, I choose to present my views as satire. I prefer poking fun and bursting balloons. I tweak myself at the same time as I kid my colleagues. After all, am I not a doctor too? Do I not exhibit the same fears, foibles and flaws? You bet I do. I know it, and my patients know it.

Many of my medical acquaintances claim that I write with a crayon because I'm so crazy I can't be trusted with pointy objects. These doctors do not find me at all amusing. In truth, my writing did get me in trouble in 1983.

I had published three columns in a row, all uncomplimentary to doctors, in the *Poughkeepsie Journal*, a daily newspaper across the state line in Dutchess County. The Poughkeepsie doctors didn't know me and they didn't appreciate my brand of humor. They made a miscalculation by formally complaining to the Litchfield County Medical Association, my home medical society, that I was being unprofessional. I got wind of the complaint and notified the editors of several local papers carrying my column. When the complaint was received in Connecticut, more than the letter hit the fan. We were ready to do battle on the basis of the First Amendment guarantee of free speech. Other papers, including *The New York Times*, picked up the David-and-Goliath story. Soon I was interviewed on local television, and later, CBS did a story on the *Evening News*.

Within weeks, the formal complaint was as uninteresting as last month's newspaper. The Poughkeepsie doctors never followed through on the complaint, the medical society took no action, and I continued to practice medicine and to write. My life changed, however. My big mouth had gained me national attention; as a result, I was able to syndicate my column nationwide. Through United Feature Syndicate, my writing is now carried daily in more than four hundred papers.

Will Rogers once said: "Everything is funny as long as it is happening to somebody else." This is certainly true of the medical profession. Any doctor can get an audience by writing about "them"—the "other doctors," the incompetents, the drug abusers, the medical crooks. I don't write about "them." I write about "us," and that infuriates some members of my profession. My purpose is to demystify. My message is: "Hey, guys, loosen up a bit. We all have problems. We're all in this together. Basically, we're all human. Sit back and have a laugh at us, at you and me. It might do you some good." I have found that ordinary people relish my irreverent barbs; so, incidentally, do some physicians, many of whom have been kind enough to write in support of my efforts.

You see, for centuries physicians have regarded themselves as privileged and unique. In every culture, consumers—the patients—have permitted a perpetuation of the mystical, miraculous and magical components of the healing arts. Medicine men, shamans and doctors have historically developed imaginative methods to maintain advantageous social and economic positions in their communities. Today we accomplish this through a powerful fraternity.

I am a member of this fraternity. I went to the "right" schools, trained in the "right" residency and am in the solo practice of medicine. I am not a young, idealistic, angry physician. But in dealing with patients and colleagues, I have come to recognize certain anachronistic tendencies that doctors exhibit. We are exclusionary. We lust after power. We behave in ways that are the very antithesis of good patient care. Arrogance and avarice threaten to undermine compassion and dedication. Obfuscation supplants teaching. The God of Science is replacing the God of Our Fathers. Although doctors *say* they care about patients, more and more patients are beginning to believe that doctors care more about themselves.

In the final analysis, physicians provide services that can easily be understood by most competent laymen. We fix things. Because of a long medical legacy, we choose to make the fixing look difficult or mysterious. Really, most of the time it is quite simple. Likewise, although diseases seem complex and unpredictable, many are relatively easy to comprehend—at least on a practical level.

Most doctors seem uncomfortable about sharing professional "secrets" with ordinary individuals. Nonetheless, people have a need to know. This need requires information and perspective. To an extent, it also involves the de-deification of the physician who is occasionally barbaric, sometimes cruel, and often downright silly. If knowledge is the bread of good health, humor must be the leavening in the loaf. The humanizing of medicine may not be around the next corner, but it is coming. An informed public, which can define and articulate what it wants, is the key.

CHAPTER 1

THE
CLUB

PERQUISITES

❖

The fledgling doctor might argue that the M.D. degree gives him a long-awaited permit to heal the sick. But such a simple view ain't, as Gershwin wrote, necessarily so. Before the young healer can put to use what he has learned, he has to become licensed in the state of his choice, obtain a job (or start his own practice), be accepted into the county medical society, qualify for malpractice insurance, be politic at the hospital to ensure a source of referrals, and—finally—trust the community he serves to support him.

Because the M.D. degree can be seen as just a step—albeit a very important one—in the development of a physician or surgeon, what exactly does the degree entitle the bearer to enjoy?

To begin with, the degree allows the bearer to obtain special license plates for his car. When attending the theater or a hockey game, the doctor can park in the most outrageous places with minimal fear of being towed away. Also, M.D. plates are, in the current vernacular, a real ego trip. They give instant status. Moreover, in consenting states, the doctor can apply for and receive tags that tout his specialty—like HEART-MD—or his name. Dr. Silverstein can thereby legally advertise as DR-SVRSTN.

Second, the M.D. degree permits the motor vehicle operator to drive at excessive speeds. Since most dangerously ill patients are being well cared for in hospital intensive care units, the doctor has no real need to speed. He drives fast because it's fun and he can always plead that he is "on an emergency." This ploy has helped innumerable physicians who, after an afternoon of golf, were late getting home for their wives' birthdays.

Third, the M.D. degree enables doctors to avoid unwanted social obligations. We are all invited to places we do not want to go to. Particularly on Tuesday night. At the Abernathys. By claiming to be "on call" or "stuck at the hospital," the doctor is in the enviable position of being able gracefully to beg out of social engagements he did not want to accept in the first place.

Fourth, the M.D. degree permits the bearer to become a member of The Club. This is not the country club—*that* can be tough enough. *The* Club: the club of doctors. Of course, once a doctor is a member of The Club, he has certain obligations. He must refer constantly to how little money he has, yet live in a large and well-appointed house; become pompous and arrogant but not speak ill of his colleagues; make sure that "his" hospital is run for the benefit of doctors, not patients; not allow patient convenience to compromise his own; never write anything that criticizes The Club. In return, the doctor will not be charged for routine medical care; can obtain enough free drugs from pharmaceutical companies to supply his own modest requirements for codeine; can drink too much, raise a little hell (when off duty) and generally indulge himself to whatever extent he pleases.

Fifth, the M.D. degree is an open invitation to borrow money without collateral. The poor slob down at the factory has to hock his car to pay for Triscuits. The doctor, on the other hand, has an unlimited line of credit; in fact, some lending agencies actually woo doctors for mortgages and that little extra cash needed for a new BMW. Friends, the M.D. degree is a license to steal. Ethan Mergatroyd can't borrow a dime; E. Mergatroyd, M.D., can write his own ticket, finance a shopping center and live well beyond his means on someone else's dough.

In referring to certain spin-offs of the M.D. degree, I realize that these misuses are the consequences of a piece of paper. After young men and women have been graduated from medical school and put up with all the bulldiddly of becoming doctors, they can still retain the dream of administering to people in need. They can be sensitive, caring and skillful. Without embarrassment and contamination of greed and power, they can

unselfishly take care of sick people and perform great deeds of
generosity. Can't they?

I CONFESS

❖

I get a kick out of doctors.

We constantly poor mouth about financial woes, high overhead and low collection rates, yet we send our children to private schools, live in big houses and drive new cars (sometimes very expensive ones).

We complain about patients' insensitivity; however, we often feel uncomfortable about empathizing with those under our care. We do not deal effectively with the deaths of our patients and the bereavements of their families. We have been taught to avoid emotional involvement, which means we may require years of experience in order to learn how to get close to people.

We gripe about our long working hours. But whenever a patient is sick, his doctor always seems to be on vacation or off duty for the weekend.

We are annoyed at having to practice "defensive medicine," but, out of curiosity, we are eager to order laboratory tests to overutilize the newest and most expensive machines and gadgets. In addition, although we are often quite correctly viewed as egocentric and irrationally independent, we are too insecure to trust our eyes and ears—our clinical judgment—in diagnosing disease. We order tests that sometimes bear no relation to the problem we are investigating. We are afraid to make mistakes and far more afraid of *admitting* our mistakes.

We hold on to patients as though they somehow belong to us by right. On the other hand, if patients cannot (or will not) follow our directions, we tell them—out of frustration—to find another doctor. We rarely take our own advice. We deny our own unhappiness; we have one of the highest rates of alcoholism, drug abuse and suicide of any profession.

We adopt the attitude that patients, families, hospital personnel, nurses—in fact most other people—are inferior. We pontificate. We are self-righteous. We deny that we are fallible, impatient, materialistic and occasionally not too bright. We cannot stand the realization that we are human and often cannot exercise the control over others—much less ourselves—that we would like.

We are often impractical. We are sometimes downright cruel. We have inflated ideas of our own worth. We pretend that we are brilliant businessmen, cagey investors, flawless parents, sources of unimpeachable truth, experts on most subjects.

We make an issue of ensuring that medical subjects and diseases are unintelligible to those not admitted to The Club. If we can't write uninterpretable prescriptions in Latin, we simply write illegibly. We find pleasing the tendency of avoiding explanations to patients, preferring instead silence or the arrogance of telling sick people that only we know what is best for them.

We demand respect without always taking the time and trouble to earn it. We are enthralled by our own perceived importance. We criticize patients for being naïve and stupid, yet we fail to make a concerted effort to instruct them about themselves, their minds and their bodies.

We have established effective methods of depreciating non-M.D. practitioners and keeping them on the fringes of the medical establishment, yet we lose millions of patients to these practitioners because we are viewed as being uncaring and ineffective. We deny that we are vulnerable.

We complain that we are always on call, but we seem to place obstacles in the way of patients who try to find us after hours. We blame patients for their diseases—because they do or do not do something—when part of the problem may be that we haven't made the correct diagnosis or suggested the proper treatment. We prescribe loads of medicine and then cluck our tongues, shake our heads and prescribe still more to counteract the side effects of the original drugs.

We have the best and the worst in our profession, but we are usually unable to tell the difference and punish the miscreants. We rage about government interference, yet most of our actions seem calculated to force government to interfere.

We tend to oversimplify. We write newspaper columns and books to see our names in print...

THE WAITING ROOM

❖

Anyone can attest to the fact that the physician's waiting room is aptly named. It's a place where you pay the doctor for the privilege of waiting... and waiting... and waiting.

I am constantly amazed to discover how much guff intelligent people will put up with. Housewives, who organize with exact precision a vacation for five family members at Cape Cod, sit for hours looking at their nail polish in these waiting rooms. High-powered, busy executives whose businesses depend on split-second accuracy for appointments and meetings cool their heels in dingy waiting rooms, haplessly checking their digital watches as precious minutes tick by. Where is the doctor? What on earth is he *doing* that is so important? Patients apprehensively lounge for hours while baby-sitters collect time and a half and harassed bank secretaries field telephone calls that the boss promised to return before 3 P.M. In what other business can you keep valued clients and paying customers waiting interminable periods? What *is* the doctor doing?

He has an emergency. Someone in greater need than you requires the unscheduled attention of the doctor. He has an emergency! Can you believe it?

Well, I don't believe it. It's pure bunk. I am going to let you in on a little trade secret. The doctor keeps people waiting because he is so disorganized that he has overscheduled himself. He is hungry to keep his office filled, and it doesn't really matter who is caught in the game—providing the doctor himself doesn't have to wait. Furthermore, he hasn't had the courtesy to allow proper time for each patient.

You see, he was already thirty-five minutes late getting to the office because he received, at the hospital, a very disturbing twenty-minute call about his stock portfolio. This was shortly followed by a fifteen-minute discussion with another doctor in the hospital parking lot about the relative merits of a Porsche 944 over a Datsun 280Z. Of course, once he arrived at the office and noted—with supreme satisfaction—that patients were starting to pile up like 747s over Kennedy Airport, he had to have a couple of telephone consultations with other doctors about sick patients. And, doctors being what they are, the talk eventually got around to golf scores and did you have a super time in St. Croix last March and how are the kids. You know, *vital* stuff. Emergencies.

So, by the time he sees his first patient, he is an hour late, and the waiting patients have long since devoured last December's *Esquire* and the most recent *Newsweek*, which is already seven weeks old. The first patient is there for a complete examination, which ordinarily takes fifty minutes. But the doctor has allowed only fifteen minutes and... well, there you are. "Yes, Gladys, he sure does keep you waiting a long time, but he must be good or he wouldn't be so busy."

I think it's about time we doctors shaped up. Let's be more aware of patients' time; it's as valuable as our own. If we really have a bona fide emergency—and they do happen—let's call the office and have our receptionists tell patients just how late we will be and offer them the option of making future appointments on a less hectic day, when they can be seen on time. Let's make an effort to adapt time slots to patients' needs. Let's stop kidding ourselves that making patients wait is a reflection of our own importance.

The next time you have an unexplained delay of more than forty-five minutes at your doctor's office, leave and send him a bill for your time. And make sure you charge the guy plenty.

FORCED FAMILIARITY

In the first scene, a young white-coated physician introduces himself to a frail elderly woman.

"Hello, Irene, I'm Doctor Williams."

In the second scene, a cheerful and crisply uniformed nurse asks a portly postoperative man: "Well, Harry, how are we today?" The nurse wears a plastic badge that identifies her as N. Pritchard.

In the third scene, a middle-aged black woman asks her gynecologist to reach under the bed for her slippers. He replies: "Come on, Gloria, you've got to get up and do these things for yourself!"

What is wrong with these three fictitious transactions? In each case, the doctor or nurse is engaging in what I call "forced familiarity," the unsolicited use of first names. This practice is engulfing the medical profession. Because its basis is destructive, we must address the issue. Forced familiarity is as much a part of the medical practice as is the rectal examination — and about as popular with patients. Did you ever ask yourself why the doctor is privileged to call you by your first name, while you are expected to call him "Doctor"?

The reason is simple. First-name calling is yet another insidious but effective way of underscoring patients' helplessness and vulnerability. It is a method by which medical people emphasize others' inferiority. We all do this with children and menial workers, often with women and the elderly. However, doctors — particularly young ones — are notorious in this regard. Although many physicians address their patients by first names out of friendship and informality, there are doctors who adopt a first-name basis in order to gain superiority.

I may be criticized for raising a nonissue—yet another unjustified attack on my worthy colleagues—but reality proves otherwise. Think of the times when you—a patient, child, woman, elderly person, or minority individual—have been called by your first name by a doctor (or nurse) you hardly knew. In return, the doctor expects to be called "Doctor" So-and-so. Last name only, please, even if the physician is young enough to be your grandson.

"Hello, Mae, how are you feeling?"

"Fine, Doctor. I'm just in for a checkup."

That dialogue may sound appropriate, but what does it mean? Mae is a seventy-six-year-old widow; the doctor is thirty-two and has just opened his practice.

I have no objection to first names, *providing* the doctor is willing to be called by *his* first name. That is the acid test. Physicians, like everyone else, prefer some degree of formality until friend-to-friend relations have been established. Jumping beyond that relation may be still another very effective method of ensuring that the doctor-patient contact remains unequal, with you know who in charge. In my opinion, forced familiarity has no place in dealing with and helping sick people.

Doctors may choose to encourage bilateral familiarity. In the final analysis, that is a question of style upon which both patient and doctor can agree. On the other hand, one-sided familiarity is condescending and patronizing.

If you don't know your doctor's first name, find out what it is before you see him . . . just in case. The next time he asks: "Well, Flora, how are things going?" answer him: "Not so good, Bill; otherwise I wouldn't be here."

Watch his eyes.

THE MASSACHU-SETTS METHOD

❖

The doctors' magazine *Medical Economics* published an article a couple of years ago by a Massachusetts internist that endorses a rather extraordinary view. It advises other physicians to fake answers to patients' difficult questions. That is, if a patient asks his M.D. a question that the doctor cannot answer, the physician is supposed to make up a response; he is never to admit he doesn't know. "Confessing your ignorance," the good doctor explains in the article, "is unfair to the patient and damn poor medicine besides."

He favors standard medical sidesteps like "temporary trouble with your circulation" and "just an exaggeration of normal functions." His prize parry is: "That's a sure sign your body is healing properly." He is a master at telling patients what they don't have, and he has developed a science of predicting what's going to happen to the symptoms of the disease he is not sure of. His final recommendations to neophyte healers are: "Watch your body language" and "schedule a follow-up visit."

I've been trying out the Massachusetts Method because patients ask hard questions, and this doctor says that if I admit I don't know the answers to the questions, the patients are likely to go down the block and find a physician who does. That could mean a drop in income, and as everybody knows, income is what keeps doctors on their toes or their mettle or whatever.

Anyway, I thought I'd follow the guy's advice. When a fortyish athletic type came into the office because of chest pains, I didn't know what was causing them. To make him feel better I told him he was just getting old and would have to learn to live with his condition. The character had the nerve to throw one of his running shoes at me.

Next, I attempted to tell a patient what she didn't have. That made sense to me, and I knew it would reassure her. She had missed her period. I wasn't sure whether or not she was pregnant, so I crooned: "Well, at least you don't have heart disease!" She refused to pay her bill and stormed out of the office.

Finally, I made an effort to predict what was going to happen. This macho kid in a motorcycle jacket thought he had VD. How could I tell without tests? But he wanted an answer. Fast. I told him: "Hang on for a few days. The symptoms may come back once or twice, or they may go away, or they may bother you, though I doubt they will." The creep walked out and had the brass to let the air out of the tires on my Porsche.

All that stuff in *Medical Economics* really didn't help me much. Maybe that Massachusetts doctor didn't go far enough. You'll be glad to learn that I've developed my own techniques, and they're foolproof.

"I've never heard of it, so it can't exist." This ploy works surprisingly well for middle-aged flower children who are into macrobiotics, massage, Zen, Zing and like that. They are usually dumbfounded at my casual frankness and amazing display of wisdom.

"It's all in your head." This never fails. I understand that this answer will fit any question and is used almost universally by all physicians, except psychiatrists. I've had great success with it. Why, just the other day I saw an old goat who was yellow as a lemon and drank a fifth a day. Poor clown may have had some cruddy disease or other, but I couldn't figure it out—it must have been in his head.

I'll bet you can improve on what I've said with your own version. Don't forget that some doctors think they should never admit there's something they don't know. The best part is that patients often have to pay for a follow-up visit to discover if the doctor's guesses were right in the first place.

**GAMES
DOCTORS
PLAY**

❖

I am sometimes frankly amazed by what passes for good medical care.

I am told that some Florida doctors, for example, accept new patients only if they agree to undergo diagnostic evaluations, including expensive examinations and laboratory screenings. A part of me wants to agree that before an elderly person is treated, a competent physician would insist on performing a thorough analysis of that patient's medical state.

But another, more practical part of me—the skeptic— understands that this approach is a lot of bull. Who needs a thorough exam to treat the myriad of minor disorders that afflict both young and old? Let's be honest, colleagues. A detailed examination, with lab work, electrocardiogram, X rays, and goodness knows what else, really serves mainly to feather the doctor's nest. This overkill technique is designed to ensure the doctor a tidy fee (to be paid largely by Medicare) and, at the same time, prevent patients with minor ailments from getting good, inexpensive care from October to May. Would you, as a sunbird, go to a doctor for swollen ankles or heartburn if you knew that such penny-ante complaints might cost you hundreds of dollars?

On a more personal note, I have a patient who seems to be intelligent, sensitive and well educated. She lives in New Jersey and has had recurring chest discomfort. Her Jersey doctor, who, for all I know, may be the greatest diagnostician since Osler, has not chosen to explain to her the possible causes of her discomfort. Rather than trying to find out what's wrong with her, he has seemingly preferred first to treat her symptoms with medicine and see how she responds.

That's not a sin; all doctors occasionally do it. However, had he shown her the courtesy of explaining what he was doing and why, she would not be confused and fearful that she might have heart disease. The definitive tests for heart problems were not immediately ordered. I am further concerned because trials of medicine can actually confuse diagnosis. Since nitroglycerin and other heart drugs often temporarily relieve the pain of ulcers and hiatal hernia, even if she improves she still won't know what is causing her problem and whether it is likely to recur or worsen.

I am not arguing against the use of trial medicine by doctors in all cases, but I do object to the tendencies of certain doctors to prescribe in a void. Physicians tend to encourage too much pill-popping anyway, without taking into account the side effects of drugs.

I also worry that what medical people tell their patients may not be "getting through." If a sick person isn't told, or doesn't understand, why something is being done, he has a right to ask and not be intimidated. The doctor, for his part, has an obligation to explain his treatment and make sure the patient plays an integral role in the decision. If not, the patient should find another doctor. Although I am not convinced that what I am told by patients about other doctors is always gospel, I am often uncertain whether their medical care is reprehensible or whether the patients *perceive* that proper care is lacking. Either way, the patient loses.

These are only some of the ways in which many—but by no means all—doctors practice a brand of medicine that although usually competent, tends to provide the greatest comfort for the physician, not the patient. This may help explain why the image of the medical profession is so tarnished today.

CHAPTER 2

DOCTORS FROM OUTER SPACE: THE MERGATROYD FILE

❖

DOCTORS FROM OUTER SPACE

❖

The classic science-fiction movie *Invasion of the Body Snatchers* depicts the horror of earth being taken over by hordes of alien plants. The intruders are devious and convincing—and therein lies the shock value of the film.

The plants produce seed pods that are capable of duplicating the characteristics of earthlings. They cover human victims with spiderwebby cocoons, and as each human dies, his plant double emerges from the cocoon and begins to function as an identical replica—with one important difference: each carbon copy has a single-minded devotion and loyalty to his leafy brethren.

You can't tell, solely by appearances, who's alien and who's human—until it's too late. To the movie's protagonists, every acquaintance is suspect; action against the invaders becomes the only way in which humanness can be determined.

I sometimes think that the film can be seen as a metaphor for the medical profession.

If you ask the average first-year medical student why he (or she) has chosen a career in medicine, he probably will respond that he feels drawn to people in need. He wants to do some good in the world; he wants to be useful.

Yet all too often, during the course of his training, he changes. I may be guilty of unfairly generalizing, but by the time he has been out of residency a while, the doctor has become a pod person. His outward human characteristics remain easily recognizable, but a disastrous and fundamental change has occurred within. Although he still talks the same way and mouths the same platitudes, inside—where it counts—he has metamorphosed into a frighteningly foreign creature.

Obviously, this progression doesn't have to occur. There are many kind, considerate, genuinely dedicated doctors around. The best physicians—and there are many—remain uncontaminated. However, along the way, our training—or the exigencies of earning a living—modify most of us. Small wonder today's doctors are viewed as arrogant and uncaring.

For a profession that has historically been obsessed with appearances, this change is puzzling. You'd expect us to make an all-out effort to maintain the image of warmth and concern that bathed and nurtured us during medical school. But often we don't. Perhaps the reason is that we voluntarily undergo paramilitary training programs that consist of exhausting, prolonged, abominably self-centering, inanely rigorous, dehumanizing, dipso-schizo boot camps.

Following this training, we strive to maintain the illusion that we compassionately serve the sick and valiantly combat disease. In reality, we often present the opposite, more accurate image. Although we are overly sensitive to appearances, we act in ways that frustrate and anger our patients, the very people we once vowed to respect, honor and help.

Patients are willing to pay a fair fee for services rendered, providing they get the service they expect. Money really isn't the issue. Doctors, on the other hand, seem increasingly oriented toward giving less and expecting more.

Have we lost sight of our original, altruistic goal? Was the goal realistic in the first place?

I believe that physicians, unlike the aliens in *Invasion of the Body Snatchers*, have the capacity to change back to their fully human selves. I am convinced that we had better exercise that capacity before we are uniformly regarded as invaders from another planet. We could start by remembering the reasons we were drawn to the medical profession in the first place, instead of behaving like a crop of pod people.

BLUE-PLATE SPECIALTY

❖

Dr. Ethan Mergatroyd gazed out of the sooty third-floor window of the staff lounge and ruminated about his future. He was completing his final year of residency at Casa Morosa General Hospital, and if he had learned anything from his training, it was that social contacts and the right specialty were the two most important determinants of success. To Ethan, success was defined as the accumulation of wealth with as little effort as possible. During his four years of medical school, followed by another four years of internship and residency, Mergatroyd had metamorphosed from an ugly caterpillar of optimistic humanism into the glorious butterfly of professional pragmatism. He would soon be ready for private practice in the real world: What should his specialty be?

He rejected a career in obstetrics because he had never been able to intimidate women in the accepted manner. He didn't like pediatrics because children frightened him. Surgery was out; he couldn't stand the sight of blood, although the money was terrific and would enable him to live out a fantasy life of conspicuous consumption. He detested internal medicine because Medicare pays less than half the doctor's fees. Likewise, geriatrics was unacceptable. Rheumatology was unattractive because he realized he certainly couldn't help anyone with arthritis. Hematology was boring. He scoffed at gastroenterologists as being "pooper snoopers." Radiologists tended to contract serious diseases because they get lazy about shielding themselves from radiation and, anyway, Ethan had never even been able to take a decent snapshot with his Instamatic. By the time pathologists dealt with people, it was usually too late. Dermatology appealed to him because patients never died, and he could charge exorbitant office fees, but he ruled out that specialty—and infectious diseases—because he found pimples and pus disagreeable. Cardiology and chest medicine were too time-consuming. Diseases of the kidneys and a specialty in metabolism were too difficult. Psychiatrists were as crazy as their patients. He was stuck. What was left?

Ethan shifted position on the plastic couch and idly watched a long, silver Mercedes pull into the doctors' parking lot. The auto slowly nuzzled into a space reserved for the handicapped, and an exuberantly healthy, immaculately dressed physician disembarked from the car. Ethan recognized him: a doctor he admired for his habit of loudly berating elderly patients waiting to be seen in the hospital emergency room. This was one doctor who never put up with the nonsense of accepting Medicare or Medicaid assignments.

Suddenly, Ethan Mergatroyd's future opened, like an Old Testament vision, before his very eyes. The choice of specialty at once became clear, as though the cobwebs of indecision had been brushed away by an unseen cosmic hand. His problem would be solved, his success guaranteed, his access to Molson's Ale and Brooks Brothers assured. In that flash of insight ordinarily reserved for mystics, Ethan's path was made clear to him: he would enter medicine's newest specialty, Diseases of the Rich.

It is beyond the scope of this report to describe the intricacies of this form of medical practice. Suffice it to say that such a specialty exerts an overwhelming magnetism for today's physicians and surgeons. It is rapidly attracting more doctors. The urge to help those in need, which drew so many older, more naïve doctors to the healing profession, pales by comparison. The new specialty is here to stay, and Ethan Mergatroyd can be counted on to ride the crest of the wave. Long may he prosper.

**GETTING
A
GIMMICK**

❖

Dr. Ethan Mergatroyd was in trouble. On an overwhelming hunch, he had just pledged $10,000 for one hundred shares of an obscure electronics company. As he hung up the telephone, he remembered a trifling detail: he didn't have the $10,000 to invest.

The sinking feeling in Ethan's stomach, which was nestled behind the silk shirt deep within a forty-eight-inch waistline, soon lessened as he fantasized about the perquisites of his profession. He knew, with absolute certainty, that all doctors— and particularly himself—were destined to become experienced business tycoons. Only the poor clods whose whining articles appeared in magazines like *Medical Economics* were losers. Like others who had scratched and fought their way into a career of healing, Mergatroyd was convinced that a medical degree entitles the holder to instant business acumen and conspicuous success in the real world of finance. He needed only . . . the Big Deal.

Nevertheless, his lingering gut ache reminded him of that pesky and elusive $10,000.

How to get it? His ersatz Colonial home was mortgaged to the hilt. Monthly payments on his Mercedes Turbo were back-breaking. He had already deferred his yearly Keogh payment in order to invest in a Broadway musical about Bernhard Goetz; he had used his IRA money for a well-deserved Caribbean vacation. His alimony commitments were a hemorrhage. He leaned back in his plastic chamois chair and reflected on an event that had occurred earlier in the day.

He was driving to the office in his two-seat sports car. His golf bag was propped vertically on the seat beside him, a mute and multiheaded Gorgonian passenger. Courtesy of a traffic light,

he unexpectedly found himself in the middle of a funeral procession. As the string of cars crept along, Ethan's frustration was
exceeded only by his acute embarrassment. Was there a former
patient resting in the Slumber Wagon at the head of the line?
He really didn't want to become involved, commit to the somber
procession by turning on his headlights. Still...

He hesitated a moment, then flicked on his parking lights.
This approach seemed genteel, the right touch, the necessary
gesture in case anyone recognized his car . . . just the appropriate
method to show some respect yet achieve emotional distance—
a trait he had cultivated since serving his internship in that
steamy hospital with all its minority groups.

But he was a believer in psychic signs and wanted, at all
cost, to avoid solecism. Was the Big Chief of Staff in the sky
trying to tell him something? What would pass through the mind
of an observer witnessing a paunchy and balding Health-Care
Practitioner, with his dimmers on, chauffeuring a set of golf
clubs in a funeral procession? Maybe he shouldn't make any
big investment decisions today.

Here he was, however, his hand touching the warm telephone
cradled on his desk. He'd just spent $10,000 he didn't have.
Well, he thought, so what? Appearances are what count. The
patients are there to support the doctor, aren't they? Hadn't he
survived so far? Okay, so the Toyota dealership had been a
mistake. Everyone makes a mistake once in a while. Never go
into partnership with a lawyer. No guts. They were lucky to have
been bought out at a small loss. Computers, microchips, elec-
tronics—that's where the real money is.

The Medicare freeze had hurt. Although Ethan had jacked
up his fees in 1984, the crummy bureaucrats were still paying
him only a fraction of what he required to maintain his standard
of living.

For the thousandth time, he considered that what he really
needed was a gimmick, something in the office to enable him
to make a killing. He flinched. Poor choice of word. That was
going too far. Perhaps a little CAT scanner. True, he didn't know

how to read the pictures, but that didn't seem like an insurmountable problem. Most of the doctors who used scanners didn't know how to read them either. His thoughts trailed off as he dreamily realized he was an hour late for his first appointment.

Yep, in this business, Ethan mused, you had to have a gimmick. All that claptrap about dedication to and sacrifice for the sick was on the way out. He was repelled by illness. New doctors flocked to the ranks of jaded older physicians who relied exclusively on machines. A CAT scanner might well be the answer. Exorbitant medical fees were simply a means to hit the jackpot in the stock market. Municipal bonds were replacing the stethoscope. Tax-shelter prospectuses made much more interesting reading than medical journals and were far more useful.

Mergatroyd felt the swelling pride when he considered the exciting new world of medical practice. And he was on the cutting edge.

He resolved to borrow the $10,000, because without investments, Ethan concluded, doctors are like chickens: parts is parts.

SPREADING IT AROUND

❖

DEAR JIM:

Things aren't looking good for us farmers, as I guess you've seen if you read the newspapers. Dairy farming isn't like your job, where you sit on your behind and answer the phone, taking stock orders and like that. We had to refinance the farm to avoid selling those twenty acres of high ground to a developer. We grow the best crops there, and Martha and I love to eat lunch under the shade of the white oak during haying. Martha is feeling better after her gallbladder surgery, but we have had a lot of trouble paying our medical bills. The insurance has been real slow in coming through.

Anyway, we have had sort of a disagreement with the doctor who put her to sleep for the operation—an anesthesiologist, I think he's called. His name is Dr. Mergatroyd, and he sent us a whopping bill the day Martha got out of the hospital. We mailed the bill right off to the insurance company, but those fellows are holding up payment because Dr. Mergatroyd's fee was wrong or exceeded what they call the "customary allowance" or something.

So Dr. Mergatroyd really got on my case. His secretary called me up and threatened to report me to a collection agency if I didn't pay up right away. I told her I was waiting for the insurance, but she didn't listen, got real huffy and hung up.

I'll tell you, that burned me up. It's not like we're deadbeats, or new to town. My family's been on this farm for three generations; we're not going anywhere. And everybody in town knows that we pay our bills as promptly as we can. From what I hear, that's more than can be said for Dr. Mergatroyd.

Well, about two weeks later, I had the manure spreader out behind the tractor and I was on the main road through town, going to lay down some "cow soup" on the field I lease from George Adams. You know that old spreader sort of weaves back and forth across the road and drips a fair amount on the asphalt. I had a full load and was moving slow and dripping away like anything. The stuff in the spreader was as ripe as a tomato in August—stunk to high heaven, you might say, you being a city boy now and all.

I looked around to see if I was holding up traffic—tourists seem to like farms, but farm machinery just makes them mad—and who should I see but this Dr. Mergatroyd not ten feet behind me, in a real shiny new Porsche. I think it was one of those 944 models, not a speck of dust on it. He seemed pretty irritated at having to poke along in second gear, inhaling all those "farm-fresh" odors. But any darned fool knows you don't tailgate a manure spreader.

At any rate, I got to thinking. "That," I said to myself, "is Martha's bill he is driving down the road." I "accidentally" hit that pothole in front of Dubb's Hardware and, as quick as that, the spreader dropped about fifty pounds of manure practically in the doctor's lap. I swung a look over my shoulder and, bless me, you would have laughed to beat the band. It was what we called in the war a "direct hit." The slop had hit the road and splashed up all over Dr. Mergatroyd's spanking-clean sports car—windshield, hood, everything.

Naturally, he couldn't avoid running over it, so I peppered his undercarriage too. You remember how the muck hardens like concrete and how bad it smells in rainy weather? Even if he gets it off the chassis, it'll take him weeks to scrape it off the frame.

I smiled and waved when he finally shot past, with his windshield wipers going, but I'll bet he'll remember that afternoon for a long time to come. That car was a mess. When I got home and told Martha, I thought she was going to bust her stitches, she laughed so hard.

It's not every day you get a chance like that. I know a lot of people who would welcome the opportunity though. The bill isn't what got me. It's that the doctor was so goldarn arrogant, hoity-toity, couldn't wait for insurance to pay his bill. And that secretary of his was so darned snooty, real unpleasant. He ought to say something to her. Don't they realize patients aren't made of gold?

Well, that's the story. I thought you'd get a chuckle out of it. Reminds me of Billy Lee Marchant, the mechanic down at Henry's Garage. His doctor wouldn't make a house call on Billy's sick wife one night. About six months later, the doctor called Billy at home about 7:30 A.M. Seems he couldn't get his car started and was due on the golf course at eight. He called Billy to come and get him going.

"Sorry," said Billy, "I can't come out because I couldn't possibly take care of your problem at home. You'll have to bring the car to the shop where we can do the necessary testing and use those new electronic machines we just got in." That really stopped the doctor in his tracks, to have his own excuses turned against him.

Well, that's all for now. Give us a call next time you're up visiting your mother. Stay well,

Your friend,
ED

CHAPTER 3

M. D. DOESN'T MEAN MAGICAL DEITY

You have only to be present when Seiji Ozawa conducts the Boston Symphony in the shed at Tanglewood to appreciate that a symphony orchestra is at the pinnacle of human achievement. The organization, coordination and performance by disciplined musicians are a testimonial to our higher functioning. In no other endeavor do the parts so perfectly become the whole. I am astounded that a composer can "hear" a symphony in his head, write it out, perfect it, score it, and pass it on to a diverse and unknown group of people who, despite individual talents, interests and prejudices, will synthesize written notes into audible sequences that have the power to move us, raise us, give us beauty time after time.

What's more, this miracle is accomplished, as it has been for centuries, without microchips, video screens, assembly lines, internal-combustion engines, bathroom cleaners, fallout, plastic, preservatives, pollutants, pesticides or pizza. The amazing essence, I suppose, is that each musician subjugates his natural tendency toward independence to the complete organism of the performing orchestra. The individual artist, with beelike precision and singular purpose, contributes a well-defined part to creating something that transcends each member of the group.

Before I am dubbed a throwback to the Big Brotherism of Orwell's *1984*, let me emphasize that artistic creativity is not, for a variety of reasons, synonymous with political or industrial systems that function to control or produce, rather than to elevate, our sensibilities. In addition, I am moderately aware of the practical problems that are faced by performers in any concert hall. Nonetheless, in simplest terms, musicians in a symphony orchestra play their instruments, work together and thereby produce great beauty. I think doctors could take a cue from this spirit of collaboration.

Difficult surgery and the caring of critically ill or injured patients require enormous self-dedication as well as the coordination of massive resources. However, in other cases, doctors seem to prefer functioning in a vacuum, with inordinate reliance on technology. We doctors frequently refuse to involve other people—nurses, technicians, family members, even patients themselves—in decisions about medical care. Government agencies, insurance companies, hospital administrators, lawyers and consumers have all come to be viewed as unsympathetic to doctors or, at worst, downright antagonistic to our efforts to heal. Some doctors appear to need re-education.

You see, if the doctor is likened to an orchestra conductor (and I am being generous in that analogy), he still needs close help from ancillary professionals. To further the analogy, can you imagine the chaos that would result if the maestro failed to involve the lighting crew, the audio team or the ticket sellers, much less the musicians? How about the orchestra's trustees? The theater owner? Wardrobe? Maintenance?

Because of burgeoning medical costs and progressive tarnishing of their image, doctors might find this a good time to re-evaluate their traditional role of high priest. The M.D. degree does not mean Magical Deity. It really indicates a level of training that, through experience and many mistakes, enables the bearer to coordinate a team effort. Without the team, the doctor may find himself alone on an empty, darkened stage.

If medicine is going to survive as an honorable profession into the next few decades, we physicians had better start dealing with the reality that health care is rapidly pricing itself out of reach of all but the very poor and the very rich. It's time we began seriously orchestrating the problems we face, rather than standing on the podium before an imaginary orchestra, waving our arms to comfortingly familiar but nonexistent music.

DEITIES-
IN-
TRAINING

As I grow older, I am beginning to reflect on the interesting ways my perspective has changed. I've discovered something that happens in middle age. That something, like the squirrels that chew holes in my garden shed each autumn, is the gnawing realization that as life grows longer, death comes closer. I wonder—with some apprehension, I must admit—what diseases I am going to have to put up with... and when. I am very attuned to the elderly who, having discovered they have these diseases, face them, it seems to me, with great courage, cope with them effectively and—in many cases—conquer them.

Doctors, on the other hand, appear to be getting younger each year. And while young doctors are a resource of information, their points of view do not always match my own. These inexperienced practitioners, although they may be providing valuable services to those in middle age and beyond, often, at the same time, give us things we don't need.

For instance, we don't need to be told what to do. Many older patients are viewed by young doctors as senile, brainless inconveniences, unable to make decisions about the most fundamental issues. Therefore, the young doctor feels justified in treating them like children. This unhappy prejudice may make life much simpler for doctors-in-training, but it does little to encourage the elderly to maintain much-needed control of their lives. I would like to go on record as saying that we oldies, with a few exceptions, are quite capable of intellectual activity that— believe it or not—includes preferences about how we are treated. Please, young colleagues, make the effort to involve us in the process called the Treatment Program.

Second, we don't need to be talked down to. A condescend-

ing attitude seems to be as prevalent today as the little stethoscopes new doctors drape around their necks. If you don't
believe me, walk into a hospital—any hospital—and try to make
sense out of how you, a visitor, are treated and what you're told.
Many physicians appear actually bored by the prospect of having
to discuss illness with the uninitiated layman.

I know from experience that it's far easier to make medical
decisions about a patient without the responsibility of explanation. Whatever explanation is given may be of two kinds:
overly simplified ("Don't worry about the side effects of this
medicine") or unnecessarily obscure ("Nonsteroid agents are
more appropriate in your case because they lack hyperglycemic
and osteoporotic effects"). On occasion, "explanations" have a
decidedly ominous ring ("You'll never walk again if you don't
have this operation"). I think that we older patients are as
entitled as our younger colleagues to a reasonable and coherent
review of diseases and treatments. Please talk to us . . . not *down*
to us.

Third, we don't need a show-off. Doctors often blindly believe
in their own infallibility. The writing and publishing of case
reports and medical articles are important to a surprising number
of practitioners. But new treatments and experimental surgery
can be proved worthwhile only in human populations. That's us.
Before we consent to the investigation or treatment of symptoms,
we have to know if these modalities are generally accepted and
effective. Only then can we choose valid options and decide
whether we want to proceed. For example, coronary bypass
surgery is useful to some, but by no means to all, patients with
arteriosclerotic heart disease. Please level with us; we're grown
up enough to take it.

Finally, we don't need to have our wishes ignored. I don't
know a single person, young or old, who wants to be kept alive
indefinitely by machines, yet this subject is a major ethical and
moral dilemma in our modern society. Doctors seem to disregard
patients' beliefs in this matter. The compulsion to postpone death
has become a primary goal, almost a raison d'être, for many
practitioners. Why do doctors, young ones in particular, exhibit

such an obsession? Living Wills aside, why are we prohibited from defining the circumstances under which we will be allowed a natural death? The malpractice hooey is just a smoke screen. Families usually will welcome a reasoned approach. Please listen to us.

Treasure a physician who isn't afraid to admit he doesn't know all the answers. Canonize the practitioner who exercises common sense. Demand and expect honest communication from your doctor. If you don't like what you're hearing from him, make a fuss.

DR. FIX-IT

❖

Some families are taking a more active interest in understanding certain diseases and asking questions about the things they don't understand. I endorse this position and I believe most people feel more comfortable working *with* their doctors than being totally dependent upon them.

Predictably, not all doctors—or patients, for that matter—agree with this principle. In the June 1980 issue of the magazine *Medical Economics*, Dr. Robert Ray McGee wrote an article entitled "Patients Want to Be Their Own Doctors? Hogwash!" In the interests of fairness to an opposing view, I will summarize part of the article.

Dr. McGee quite correctly points out that the "current fad is the wellness clinics," which encourage people to abandon their bad habits, a program that the medical establishment has promoted for years. He then claims that despite dieting, jogging, and avoidance of tobacco and alcohol, "there will still be a lot of diseases you won't be immune to, including coronary artery disease." That conclusion is not valid. Risk factors do play an important role. If moderate living habits can help, I'm all for them.

The doctor also claims that when he tries to teach patients about their illnesses, they "don't hear a word you've said. It's the same as when I take my car to the garage. I have a mild interest in what the mechanic says is wrong with it, but I'm not much interested in a detailed lesson on how to fix it myself. What I want him to do is get the lemon running again. Patients aren't interested in my role as a teacher; they don't want to be taught how to take care of their bodies. They just want me to 'fix it.'"

I don't know what kind of luck Dr. McGee has with his automobiles. Probably not so good. But I cannot believe that people refuse to learn ways to improve their health. Maybe I'm naïve. I persist in the prejudice that the act of explaining health problems to patients and answering their questions has a therapeutic effect—that of increasing the teamwork and understanding between patient and doctor. I might add that most doctors I admire hold the same view. I think that patients deserve the respect of being listened to and having their difficulties discussed. In addition, when patients become more knowledgeable about disease, they can take better care of themselves. Again, there are symptoms and signs that cannot be ignored or self-treated. There is simply no excuse for anyone to ignore, for example, severe chest pains or any significant change in body function.

No, Dr. McGee. I'm afraid you're missing a very important point. People are not ignorant by choice. They need to know about what ails them. The fact that your teaching technique is apparently unsuccessful may reflect more on you than on your patients.

By the way, did you ever ask your garage mechanic whether you were doing something wrong to your poor old car to prevent its efficient operation? I can hear those mechanics laughing all the way to the bank every time you pay them to realign the wheels on the "Caddy" because your daughter keeps hitting the curb when she drives the "lemon" into the driveway.

BEST
FOR THE
PATIENT?

❖

Doctors are believed. More important, doctors believe they are believed.

This state of affairs may not be in the best interests of the patient.

Once upon a time—before antibiotics, microsurgery and a veritable armamentarium of medical treatments —doctors had relatively inconsequential therapy to offer the sick. For example, the following scene has been immortalized in a plethora of sentimental Victorian paintings: the all-knowing physician sits by the bedside of a critically ill child, earnestly straining through sheer willpower to save a life, patiently waiting for the disease to follow the traditional pattern of lysis or crisis.

Doctors were supposed to be experts on death. So their pronouncements had a magical quality, almost like a deific decree. They were not questioned, because, in large part, society put a premium on knowledge; these learned and compassionate men did what they could, under the circumstances. However, scientific medicine was yet to be "discovered." More often than not, medical management involved giving simple support and care to the family. What little knowledge medical men possessed was respected. A successful doctor was usually judged more by his ability to predict an outcome than to influence it.

Now that is no longer the case. We have CAT (CT) scanners, chem screens, chemotherapy, cryosurgery and a seemingly inexhaustible array of spanking-clean complicated machines that save lives—but at the same time probe and poison us. No longer satisfied with just helping the sick, doctors prolong, and prolong, and prolong the lives of some patients to the point where these unfortunate victims of medical know-how become social, as well as medical, problems.

I am not suggesting that modern gadgetry is not a blessing. Millions of patients are alive today because scientific advancements have enabled doctors to ameliorate suffering and cure diseases that years ago would certainly have been fatal.

Yet what are the trade-offs? Doctors are still treated as all-knowing and are believed when they say you will get well. Don't worry; leave the decisions to us; you'll feel better tomorrow. All too often, patients recognize these reassurances as falsehoods but suspend their common sense and testing of reality—with disastrous results. We're not as smart as we would like our patients to think we are. In our scramble to prolong life, we often behave in ways that minimize our own discomfort about suffering, illness and death. We are frequently less than truthful with patients, and we excuse our dishonesty by saying it is "best for the patient," when, in fact, the fraud may be our means of protecting ourselves. Finally, we cover up when we don't know the answers.

Although there are no good ways to be sick, some ways are better than others. Often, if a doctor is truthful to his sick and dying patients, the burden of illness can be lessened. Because a sick person feels helpless and vulnerable, he is usually reluctant to ask questions of those caring for him. This is not a good arrangement. Patients have a right to know what is in store for them, what is *really* the matter with them, what methods are proposed for diagnosis and treatments—and why.

Many doctors make a real effort to deal honestly with people under their care. Alas, there are still physicians who are threatened by patients who ask reasonable questions and expect reasonable answers. Often these doctors are extremely uncomfortable with their own feelings concerning illness and death; often they worry a great deal about their own potential inadequacies. They need to be educated by their patients, who in turn need to stop perceiving them as deities.

GOSPEL

Images in medicine are more complex than those black-and-white patterns seen on X-ray films that radiologists shuffle around. It is said that the entire image of American medicine is being tarnished. The crisis has reached Epidemic Proportions. There is a great hue and cry being raised by the medical guilds—the academy of this or the college of that. Doctors are viewed by the public as being no more ethical than used-car salesmen and—heaven help us—attorneys. What can be done to reverse this trend?

Good question. As a start, you must realize that people's deprecation and defilement of doctors are not the fault of the practicing physician. He or she has recognized for centuries that appearances are the very lifeblood of the profession. Therefore, most M.D.s have developed a system of plausible excuses to explain away, in wonderfully magical terms, what is perfectly apparent: namely, that doctors suffer from and exhibit the same little quirks affecting any taxpaying adult.

I've invented ten excuses and would like to try them out on you. See if you can sympathize with the overworked professional who uses them.

1. The best excuse for driving an expensive automobile: "Because of my on-call schedule, I do a lot of driving and I need a reliable car."

Next best excuse: "My brother-in-law owns the dealership."

The truth: "It's fun and makes me feel important."

2. The best excuse for raising fees: "My malpractice premiums have quadrupled."

Next best excuse: "I'm keyed into the Consumer Price Index."

The truth: "I need the extra money to pay for my new Mercedes Turbo." (See #1, above.)

3. The best excuse for not returning a patient's telephone call: "I tried, but the line was busy."

Next best: "I had an emergency."

The truth: "I forgot."

4. The best excuse for a bad reaction to prescription medicine: "I didn't know you were taking vitamins! Why didn't you tell me?"

Next best: "The pharmacist must have made a mistake."

The truth: "I didn't think of it."

5. The best excuse for the patient's condition worsening in the hospital: "The medicine didn't work."

Next best: "The nursing care was lousy."

The truth: "I didn't make the correct diagnosis."

6. The best excuse for a surgical mishap: "I didn't do it."

Next best: "It must have been my assistant."

The truth: "I got lost in there."

7. The best excuse for a padded bill: "The patient was very sick, so I had to charge more."

Next best: "My accountant [or computer] made a mistake."

The truth: "I thought I could get away with it."

8. The best excuse for not being available on Wednesday: "I was taking an advanced course at the medical center."

Next best: "I had an illness in the family."

The truth: "Wednesdays are national holidays for doctors, and I was off playing golf."

9. The best excuse for not being available at 9 P.M.: "I had a meeting."

Next best: "I've just changed my answering service."

The truth: "I was watching a good movie on TV and couldn't be bothered."

10. The best excuse for the crazy 2 A.M. order given over the telephone to the floor nurse: "I was sick with the flu and don't remember being awakened."

Next best: "I'd put in a long day and was tired."

The truth: "I drank too much brandy after dinner."

Of course, this brief sampling could be expanded to cover several more pages. My purpose is to show that we doctors are doing our darndest to improve our public images by telling people what we know they want to hear. Only the most hardened, belligerent and unsympathetic skeptic would fail to believe us. After all, physicians' statements are taken as gospel, right?

LETTING DOWN THE BARRIERS

I was rocked back on my heels the other day when a friend, in commenting about my writing, stated that it reveals a good deal about me. After a decent interval of apprehension stemming from my fears of self-revelation, I cautiously read through my stash of past articles. They dealt with a wide range of topics: witch doctors, fairy tales, doctors in general, an obituary to a colleague, questions of aging and dying. Yes, I had to agree; I am, to an extent, revealed in these articles. And, I concluded, showing myself in my writing isn't a bad thing, not a bad thing at all.

You see, the practicing physician demands that patients bare themselves. I don't mean just by physically disrobing. The doctor must learn all he can about his patients; this very privileged and confidential information is critical in enabling him to diagnose and treat illness. However, that litany—the so-called medical history—is strictly one-sided. The doctor is not about to volunteer personal items about the vicissitudes of his own life. If he is good, he asks questions about patients' fears, mistakes, fantasies, shames—in short, all the undercover elements that most people try to hide from the world.

For his part, the physician is expected to sit back and assimilate these secrets without getting involved. In fact, he is trained to avoid involvement. So he presents an image of a well-integrated, nonjudgmental healer. That image, that role, may be unrealistic to the extent that it encourages patients to perceive doctors as nonhuman and all-powerful.

However, the best doctors are not necessarily the ones who are the most aloof. Physicians often require years of experience before they can overcome the well-ingrained techniques of distancing themselves from patients, before they can say: "Yes, I know how you feel." And mean it. Therefore, the willingness of doctors to let down barriers not only reaffirms their humanness but gets them closer to patients. I believe that in a world of high tech, this welcome tendency should be encouraged. Too many physicians today are risking being viewed as just so many bright-eyed, fleshy extensions of the medical machines they seem to worship.

CHAPTER 4

CELEBRITY DOCTORS, MEDIA MEDICINE

HUMANA
OR
INHUMANA?

❖

Nothing in recent medicine has so captured the imagination of the public and the attention of the media as the medical drama of the artificial heart. Since beginning his artificial-heart program with the Humana organization, Dr. William C. DeVries, who from all accounts appears to be a first-rate surgeon with excellent technical ability, has enjoyed international recognition. But the results of his first operations in this new area of medicine have been sobering.

Barney Clark was the first. He died.

William Schroeder was the second. He was permanently braindamaged and he died in August 1986.

Murray Haydon, the third, died this year after having required a long period of post-operative hospitalization.

Jack Burcham died ten days after receiving his artificial heart in April 1985.

Thus far, the Humana artificial-heart team is not off to a propitious start. To begin with, there have been from the start some questions about the kind of consent form the four Humana patients signed. The document was said to be seventeen pages long, which seems to indicate more complexity than the average sick patient can grasp. Maybe that doesn't matter. According to newspaper reports, when questioned about the operative consent, Dr. DeVries stated that the patients ". . . told me in their own way that they don't care if they read it or not . . . they were not really interested in listening to the long list of horrors that could happen. They didn't want to hear that they may have a stroke and be unable to use all mental capabilities. Those are issues that they would rather be left unsaid."

I find this curious. In my experience, most patients facing

surgery want everything said, particularly the part about risks. Under these circumstances, most adults would like to know what is in store for them. Although Dr. DeVries' patients were, in a devastating sense, terminal, I cannot believe they were so desperate that they refused to consider the possibility of a vegetative existence.

I would not want to agree to a prolonged and agonizing death, nor would I choose to become a permanent burden on my family. I don't think I'm unique in this prejudice; many people I know express the same feelings. Are seriously ill heart patients so different? I doubt it. I think the artificial-heart recipients and their families were caught up in the ballyhoo and hype of the whole awesome mystique of the Great Experiment. Out of his own commitment to destiny, the cardiac surgeon may have been unreceptive to the fundamental decisions all of us, at one time or another, will have to make.

I hate to admit it, but we doctors can force patients to do what we want them to do. For instance, if I have a patient with terminal cancer, I have two choices: help him with the difficult process of dying or, through a subtle form of coercion, raise his hopes that treatment—any treatment—will be effective. If my reputation or my ego or my bank loans are at stake, and if I need a subject for an experiment, you can be assured I'm not going to make my patient comfortable and let him die in peace.

There is a terrible conflict of interest here, and I believe the medical community is just beginning to grapple with the hideous realization that what is best for the patient may not always be best for the doctor. We—doctors and laymen—need to ponder the ethical considerations of an M.D. who has convinced himself that artificial survival serves primarily to accelerate medical progress, benefit civilization or—from a purely practical standpoint—further his own career.

It's scary to acknowledge that some day all of us may find ourselves in potential conflict; our comfort and survival may ultimately rest in the hands of doctors whose primary commitment is to themselves.

This departure from Hippocrates has recently been addressed in the medical literature as the "not-on-my-shift" syndrome. Apparently, surgical residents in university teaching hospitals will do everything in their power to keep patients alive—until another resident arrives for the next shift. The reason? When the patient dies, it means more paper work, a covert admission of physician "failure" and a "black mark" against the resident.

We need to remind ourselves that "mercy" isn't synonymous with "at the mercy of." Technical ability is not the sole prerequisite of a good doctor.

I'm not necessarily suggesting that Dr. DeVries and his team are insensitive to or unaware of their roles in serving the sick, with the patient's best interest as their foremost goal. I'm just raising questions. In the unlikely event that I chose to be critical, I might be tempted to ask if it's true, as has been reported, that Dr. DeVries burned the diary he kept while Barney Clark was alive—and why.

MEDICINE'S TRIUMPH— BABY FAE'S PAIN

❖

More than a year after the futile attempt in 1984 to save a dying infant by implanting a baboon's heart into her chest, the *Journal of the American Medical Association* editorialized that the effort was doomed to failure from the start. The doctors at the Loma Linda University Medical Center in California who experimented on the infant—whom the world came to know as Baby Fae—were subject to "wishful thinking," according to the *Journal.*

Doctors and laymen alike appreciate the fact that the implantation of a baboon's heart into a human infant must surely rank as one of the century's most astounding technical accomplishments. But many of us felt from the very beginning that the outcome for Baby Fae was sadly predictable.

She underwent a painful, hazardous and drastic operation. Despite the use of powerful drugs to alter her immunity, her body was programmed to reject the primate heart as a foreign substance. Experience has shown that similar cases have a maximum survival of only weeks. She never really had a chance.

So all the talk we heard at the time of the operation about baboons living fifty years, and will Baby Fae be ridiculed in school, was a cruel fantasy. There was never much possibility that this unfortunate youngster would get out of diapers, much less kindergarten. I wonder what imperative caused Fae's parents to allow her to be subjected to such pain in return for a short and uncomfortable life.

Baby Fae was, for obvious reasons, unable to participate in decisions about her own future. When medical experimentation is carried out on humans—and make no mistake, Baby Fae's surgery was an experiment—we Americans have correctly demanded informed consent. Experiments on unwilling subjects in Nazi Germany are too recent a memory to be forgotten or ignored.

Legal issues of consent aside, do you for one minute assume that the Loma Linda surgeons plainly outlined to Baby Fae's parents the extent of the suffering the baby would undergo as a direct result of the surgery? To my knowledge, none of the members of the operating team had ever had open-heart surgery. How could they assess, in a meaningful way, the extreme discomfort of incisions, chest tubes, respirator, constant noise— in short, all the characteristics of a postoperative patient in an intensive care unit? Before her death, our own prematurely born daughter went through it all, and we lived it with her. We remember.

I am still concerned about the public relations aspect of the whole show. Many heart surgeons appear to need recognition and reputation as much as their patients need new hearts. It's often part of the personality of doctors who choose this dramatic specialty. Hospitals, too, require recognition. A big media blitz certainly isn't going to hurt an Adventist medical center.

The whole affair had the aura of a combination space launch and carnival, with both hospital and doctors getting prime-time, front-page publicity, while Baby Fae remained anonymous. Like Parkland Hospital in Dallas, Loma Linda will be remembered— for a different reason.

Whether medical experimentation upon human infants could be classed as child abuse is an issue I will leave to the moralists. Baby Fae, along with other heart-transplant recipients, will enter the history books. Will her sacrifices be justified by further improvements in medical technology? Perhaps. But whatever the answers to these painful questions, I am haunted by the fact that she was a vulnerable little packet of life who was pushed into taking a greater burden than most adults ever carry. One could argue that her interests would have been better served if, at birth, she had been made comfortable and her parents allowed to grieve.

We might be tempted to give scientific investigators this message: Until you get it right, pick on someone your own size.

THE OLD WAY IS STILL THE SAFEST

❖

Once upon a time, there was a Boston doctor who was interested in curing a certain form of heart disease by using a delicate operation. No one had ever operated in quite this way before, but the surgeon was optimistic that his daring technique had the potential for saving many lives. So he began by working in a laboratory with dogs.

After two trying years, he had ironed out most of the wrinkles and he wrote a short report on his findings.

The report was published by an obscure journal of experimental medicine. Other surgeons who read of the experiment attempted to duplicate the findings.

Meanwhile, the doctor continued to operate on dogs. He streamlined the surgery, defined the indications for it and made alterations that improved the success rate.

At the same time, a French surgeon—also working with dogs—verified the operation's beneficial effects. A Danish doctor reported that, in his hands, the procedure was a failure, and he discarded it. However, a group of scientists in England carefully reviewed the Danish data and concluded that the Scandinavian study had omitted a seemingly inconsequential step; this appeared to explain why the Danish doctor had failed. Once the British report was published, several surgical teams in other countries—notably Japan and South Africa—operated on monkeys and achieved conspicuous successes.

During an interval of about four years, the Boston surgeon perfected the procedure and performed it on more than fifty dogs; forty of them lived and did well. An international surgical academy invited him to present his findings at a convention in San Francisco. This he did. In his paper, he acknowledged that he had incorporated several Japanese modifications so that his stunning success was due not only to his skills but to the alternatives developed by his Asian colleagues.

Upon his return from the convention, the doctor was asked to examine a hospital patient who was dying of untreatable heart disease. She had been given two months to live, and her physicians had concluded that although the new operation had not yet been performed on humans, it might save her. The surgeon agreed.

The patient was given a concise description of the surgery, its risks, expense and possible complications. After two days of deliberation, she signed a consent form, indicating her awareness of the experimental nature of the operation and her willingness to proceed.

There was no press release.

The surgery was unobtrusively carried out; the woman recovered uneventfully and was able to live a normal life. She was never interviewed on television news. In fact, she requested that her name not be publicized, to protect her family's privacy.

During the next year, the surgeon performed his new procedure on ten other terminal cardiac patients. Eight lived, one died of pneumonia, one succumbed to kidney failure. The surgeon documented these cases in detail, and his report was published in a well-known and widely read surgical journal.

Upon publication of the report, the media became aware of the breakthrough; as a result, the doctor enjoyed much recognition and fame. His hospital became the mecca for other surgeons who adopted the procedure, and after several years, the technique became commonplace and was accepted throughout the world.

I have invented this fictitious vignette to show how, in a general way, new treatments used to become available. In essence, they were tested, retested, checked and rechecked, and—eventually—reported in reputable scientific publications. *Then* the news media were informed.

Not so now. Today, everything is backwards. A surgeon can, at a moment's notice, get full TV coverage—and relish it—while he performs a procedure that's not fully tested or safe or expected to be successful. Hardly a day passes when you can't pick up a newspaper, thumb through a newsmagazine or flick on your TV and discover the novel things doctors are doing to people. This hype really gets our hopes up, and, unfortunately, these outrageous procedures rarely succeed. How could they? They haven't been thoroughly tested, and their supposed benefits haven't been confirmed.

This whole crummy situation is not the fault of the reporters. After all, they're out there to gather news. No, the problem lies with publicity-seeking doctors and inhumane hospitals that can't wait to see their names in lights and to make lots of money.

In my view, before one word of baboon-heart transplantation was muttered to the press, the procedure should have been checked out rationally, quietly and privately—until the evidence proved it worthwhile. We still don't know its benefits or whether it is an appropriate method.

We don't even know if coronary-artery bypass surgery is effective. We're beginning, at last, to learn—a little late, I'm afraid, now that thousands of patients have undergone the operation.

I believe we have to return to a process called "scientific scrutiny." It may take a little longer to decide which new treatments are best, but, in the long run, the public will be better protected and better served. To accomplish this goal, some doctors and hospitals need to develop a quality they demand of their patients: patience.

SOME DOCTORS SELL THEIR SOULS

❖

Everyone needs a little recognition. It adds spice, like a hint of garlic in a good salad dressing. We're active in school and community affairs, in our business and social lives, and on the golf course, to obtain, among other objectives, recognition.

To one extent or another, we often gain recognition by advertising. This can take the form of assuming positions of responsibility, the ways in which we dress and talk, the types of products we consume. In moderation, advertising probably is a universal and harmless activity.

However, like garlic in salad dressing, it can be overdone. Race cars are plastered with stickers touting various companies. Professional athletes wear equipment weighted down by crisply lettered, camera-ready names of manufacturers. Even automobile makers attach visibly distinctive company initials to their products, both front and back. In an age when all cars look alike, I suppose this practice has merit when, in traffic, you're cut off by some kid in a Ford van. At least you won't blame the Chrysler Corporation for your moment of anger. Perhaps vehicle buyers should have to demonstrate safe-driving skills before the dealer rewards them by attaching the manufacturer's emblem. But I digress.

Until recently, doctors—who, God knows, crave recognition—were prohibited from advertising. There was good reason for this proscription. It was considered unprofessional for members of the healing arts; consumers were expected to judge doctors' abilities by therapeutic results, not by media bombardment. Like supporters of public television, doctors were permitted to provide their names and specialties, but no commercial messages, please.

Now all that has changed, and, like the aforementioned overspiced salad dressing, it leaves a bad taste in the mouth and can cause heartburn. The healing arts have been transformed by marketing technology into just another commodity.

I think it's fair to call the practice "unscrupulous" when certain physicians pay public relations firms thousands of dollars a month to sell the doctors as commodities. I regularly receive mailings, complete with eight-by-ten glossies, that are nothing more than promotional brochures, dreamed up by admen, for dermatologists and plastic surgeons.

Other doctors now talk to newspapers and magazines to hawk their wares. Do you enjoy watching medical "experts" on television news and talk shows? How do you think they get there? Because they're acknowledged leaders in their specialties? Not on your scalpel. There are a few exceptions, but most of the guys have paid plenty to an agent or P.R. firm to obtain the TV spot. They want media exposure, and short of shooting their mothers-in-law in time for the 7 P.M. news, this is the way to get it.

I'm convinced that such unprofessional conduct reflects a growing malignancy in the health-care system. Seattle's Dr. Thomas Preston, a writer and critic of medical materialism, dubs this blight "medical entrepreneurship": the belief that financial success is what doctoring is all about and that business marketing techniques are the way to achieve this goal.

Before hoisting myself on my own petard, let me point out the obvious: There are physicians who happen also to be athletes, artists, missionaries, businessmen, authors, inventors and social reformers. I don't think that dual-career doctors should be prohibited from promoting their nonmedical objectives. In fact, their publicity might be encouraged, because they add another dimension to a profession that often is viewed as narrowly secular.

However, I draw the line at doctors who advertise to sell their medical skills and collect new patients. Entrepreneurship appears to be a thriving ethic among young M.D.s in residency programs, and I'm concerned that this voracious behavior eventually will become the norm, rather than just a sad aberration.

The courts have established clearly that doctors who advertise are breaking no law. Nonetheless, I believe that the overwhelming majority of physicians still cherish the traditional values of professionalism, one of which I would summarize as follows: Medicine is an honorable life's work for which doctors have the right to be remunerated. Our primary goal, however, is to serve our patients, not to become rich at their expense.

Because physician advertising has no other goal but to increase earnings, I continue to believe that people will reject Madison Avenue medicine, ignore the entrepreneurs and insist on obtaining care from the type of practitioner who is, quite simply, just a good doctor.

WHY WERE WE CALLING DR. KILDARE?

❖

Television programs about doctors and hospitals have been consistently popular sources of entertainment. The public's preoccupation with things medical has its roots, I am told, in the fascination with which the average citizen views the mystical workings of a profession that we, the doctors, have purposely chosen to keep secret. We have acquiesced in this fantasy and, in turn, become its victims. By embracing the image as the reality, we have helped increase public expectations of a larger-than-life medical profession. Because no doctor could possibly live up to the television ideal, public confidence becomes eroded.

It all began when clever scriptwriters and producers discovered that the public's urge to learn more about the real world of medicine could be translated into a highly lucrative market, provided the material was dramatized and sensationalized.

For example, I can tell you there is nothing romantic about being awakened from a sound sleep at 3 A.M. to be told by the emergency room nurse that a local female alcoholic is in DT's and has been brought to the hospital for detoxification, so, Doctor, please get down here and handle it. That's the way the scene usually plays in real life. However, on TV, this comes off as a surgeon's drunken wife who went on a bender because her son contracted AIDS after being taken as a lover by the hospital's esteemed Chief Pathologist, who himself has been suspected by the Operating Room Supervisor of dealing cocaine to a promiscuous unwed mother whose former boy friend has been blackmailing the Head Dietitian, who was involved in an underground railroad for illegal Nicaraguan refugees who brought in the AIDS in the first place. And we're off and running, if you see what I mean. It goes on and on. Viewers lap this stuff up and tune in every day to see how each snarled knot of entanglement is going to be unraveled. Television's depiction of the medical world is, in the main, as inaccurate as its other soap operas, which purport to expose, for example, the private lives of Texas oil tycoons.

Sure, I'm willing to concede that this is harmless entertainment with no pretense of verisimilitude. People need this kind of escape, and powerful unions, like law and medicine, make tempting vehicles for adult fairy tales.

However, the situation isn't always so clear, is it? There are several medical hits running now, and they all give the appearance of mirroring Medical Reality. The kind, wise, principled, responsible, harassed, dedicated physician—graying at the temples, no fooling around, disdaining alcohol and drugs—is marvelously oblivious of fees, malpractice premiums, tax shelters, write-offs, investments, IRAs and no-load government bonds. He has a perfect image. He is what people want doctors to be.

The problem is, we're not. And patients are often understandably disappointed, consciously or unconsciously, when we don't live up to this appearance of perfection. Of course, we—the profession—have acquiesced in the creation of the Kildares, the Ben Caseys and all the other idealized boob-tube physicians. We helped create them, because in the medical world, as in mating rituals, display is what really counts.

We refuse to quit bragging about the marvelous accomplishments of the twentieth-century science of which we are a part. We insist on projecting the mien of the consummate old-fashioned country doc who was always available and knew what to do, when, in truth, we don't often behave like him. We like to think we have our own brand of the Right Stuff that we secretly believe makes us superior beings. But our actions belie this prejudice. Although we hunger to be perceived as ideal healers, our humanness dogs us like late-afternoon shadows.

We mendaciously portray ourselves as gentle and caring when it's perfectly obvious to any intelligent layman that we are, after all, flawed and have the same mundane concerns that characterize any sane adult in our complex society. We tend to complain about the chimera of TV doctors, but we helped create the illusion and we're now stuck with having to live up to it.

What an intolerable burden.

I think our lot would be a happier one if we could be more open and sharing, if we were more willing to demystify medical practice. I believe we need to admit our limitations, let people know our weaknesses as well as our strengths. I am convinced medicine would take a giant step forward if its practitioners could let down their hubris and help patients develop reasonable and realistic expectations about doctors' skills. Self-honesty could go a long way toward resolving the incompatibility between real doctors in a real world and professional actors in imaginary stories. Perhaps in the future, the public will come to understand that TV doctors are nothing more than amusing counterfeits bearing little resemblance to the genuine article.

TV COMMERCIALS AND OTHER FAIRY TALES

❖

We are at the mercy of our children's stories. They give us several important messages: good will triumph over evil; if you say the right things and do what is expected, you will win out; unhappiness can be overcome; goodness is always rewarded; be patient in order to succeed. In short, by behaving in certain ways, you can control your life.

Analyze any fairy tale. Almost without exception, the protagonist (you) is good, generous, trustworthy, loving, honest, loyal and misunderstood. You have a problem, usually caused by a spell or other unfortunate incident, which makes you poor, ugly or disinherited. By means of magic (a good person in your life) or hard work, you can overcome the antagonist (society, a wicked stepmother, the forces of evil). In the end, you will succeed and

live happily ever after—with love, friends, respect and wealth.
Is this the way life is? Not on your enchanted castle. However, at a primitive level we all continue to believe the myth that through our actions we can somehow control our destinies.

Never mind the children's stories we have grown up with. Look at the television commercials that bombard us. If you smell bad, don't have enough money, can't keep your floor clean, won't use the right bathroom tissue, have halitosis or gray teeth, are constipated, don't eat properly, or have hemorrhoids, you are temporarily under a spell. It can be banished by deodorants, loans, floor wax, soft toilet paper, mouthwash, laxatives, bran flakes, or Preparation H. And there's more: You also have to drive the appropriate automobile, live in the correct house, wear the proper clothes, use the best perfume and drink the right beer.

If you think I am exaggerating, pay close attention to what commercials are saying. You are unattractive (poor, misunderstood, exploited), but by behaving in a specific way (using magic) you can become beautiful and successful. A fairy tale? You bet. But we fall for it every time.

There are people in many parts of the world who are concerned with only one basic goal: survival. There are others, usually more affluent, who think that our existence is arbitrary and our fate often absurd. When they are warm and their bellies full, they read books by Sartre and Kierkegaard.

I don't believe we have to be existentialists to appreciate that life is as arbitrary as a traffic light and that our actions do not necessarily influence our ultimate happiness. But it helps.

I have patients who knowingly and systematically abuse themselves with drugs and alcohol, smoking and overeating. The payoff in their script may be death; if not, perhaps they are waiting for someone to break the evil spell so that they can be normal. After all, you have to kiss a lot of frogs before you find a prince. Patients' actions, in a very negative way, obviously influence their lives.

However, I also have patients who live exemplary lives of moderation and who get very sick, and no one understands why—because we are taught that if you do the Right Thing, you are *supposed* to get a payoff of happiness and health. We are programmed by children's stories, advertising and television to believe that everything is going to turn out all right. But it doesn't, does it? Wonderful children still get leukemia. Wonderful grandparents, with hearts of iron, are confined to nursing homes because of advanced mental decay. Wonderful fathers who jog and disdain cigarettes have massive, fatal heart attacks. Wonderful people are hurt, maimed or killed every day despite the fact that they are cautious, frugal and abstemious.

What are we to do? Keep trying, I guess. And, maybe, stop kidding ourselves that we can figure it all out. Did you ever reflect on what surprising consequences and unpleasant experiences Cinderella had *after* marrying the prince? Was she bored to tears? Was the act of acquiring the prince more enjoyable than actually having him? Perhaps she deserved what she got.

Unfortunately, fairy tales seldom tell us how to cope with life as it is; nor do they instruct us how to deal with success. Neither do television commercials. We seem to be a society with a unique compulsion to achieve success without really knowing what to do when we get there.

FATAL ERROR

❖

Bob East had just retired as a skillful and respected photographer for the Miami *Herald* when his tragic death in early 1985 made news across the nation. He entered Jackson Memorial Hospital in Miami for surgery, was inadvertently injected with a highly toxic substance, and died. The toxin had been stored in an unmarked container and wasn't supposed to be present in the operating room—but it was. And somehow, inexplicably, a nurse drew up the solution and administered it to East.

The surgeons and the hospital immediately admitted the mistake, and now all hell has broken loose. It has meant a field day for lawyers. One trial lawyer claimed—among other things— that the doctors admitted responsibility only because they found it impossible to lie. He labeled the incident tragic proof that doctors lie (when they can get away with it), falsify records, cover up mistakes and fail to discipline colleagues.

The attorney's broadside against the medical profession reflected a great deal of rage and indignation. Predictably, the lawyer's barrage also served to close medical ranks. Florida doctors united and fought back with a counterattack against the legal fraternity and their contingency fees.

All this may make sensational material for newspaper readers, but the information is hardly enlightening. It produces, as the saying goes, more heat than light.

Bob East can never be brought back. His family can never be emotionally or financially compensated for the loss of a beloved husband and father. An incomprehensible mistake was, in fact, made. The whole affair will probably be aired in a public courtroom, and—once the dust is settled—heads will roll; the East family will become wealthier, the lawyers will collect their fees, and Florida medicine will return to business as usual. Of course, the Easts will never forget, nor will the surgeons, nurses and hospital personnel.

For me, the most intriguing aspect of the newspaper reactions in Miami and elsewhere was the undeniable mistrust—even hatred—that seemed to exist between doctors and lawyers. The articles and letters appeared to highlight a brutal polarity between the two professions. This polarity is legendary and forms the basis for many amusing jokes and much friendly jousting. But East's death provoked a surprisingly violent antagonism. Perhaps it's more accurate to speculate that the antagonism has always been present and that the Miami incident simply brought it to a flash point.

In any event, I'm sorry about the viciousness. Most attorneys I know, like most doctors, are competent people who attempt to serve their clients. It seems to me that life is difficult enough without our compulsion to go at each other with fists flying. I enjoy working with lawyers for the benefit of our mutual client-patients. Of course, I disagree with many things that lawyers do, as I also disagree with doctors, dentists and the guy who drove a truck over my flowers after chipping brush. There are malevolent forces—conscious and unconscious—in every line of work, and I'll wager that good landscape gardeners have as much difficulty as good doctors and good lawyers when it comes to weeding out incompetents.

For many of us, patience and forgiveness often appear to be unattainable goals. Yet, in our complex society, events have a tendency to go wrong, and, given enough time, we are all guilty of carelessness and mistaken judgment. I object to willful negligence when, at times, professionals intentionally behave in ways that harm, exploit or depreciate others. Nothing can ever alter the awful finality of what happened to Bob East. But I cannot believe that his untimely death was due to anything more than unintended human error. With respect to attorneys who make proverbial hay under the sun of tragedy, I suggest they consider developing two characteristics that all of us—particularly lawyers—would do well to covet: compassion and humility.

CHAPTER 5

THE GALL-BLADDER IN 803

BEDPAN POWER

❖

The bedpan is a hundred-year-old contrivance that has, unfortunately, undergone few design changes during the century it has been used in hospitals. Doctors have not traditionally devoted long hours to analyzing or debating the phenomenon of the bedpan—until they, as patients, are expected to use one. Then all hell breaks loose. However, after an appropriate interval of several months, we conveniently "forget" how uncomfortable the device is and continue to insist that our patients be wedded to it.

I've often considered the old metal bedpan to have more esthetic than practical value. It seems to me that the cold, shallow, scalloped contraption would be ideal for sliding on snowy hills (like metal trays) or as containers for exotic houseplants. Maybe, in fact, the thing has no esthetic value at all; but it is shiny and smooth and makes a glorious sound when, empty, it is dropped onto a hard floor. The plastic bedpan attains no prestige whatsoever and is not even a suitable topic for discussion. It may be warmer to sit on, but it has no more appeal than tacky, modern, rubberized automobile bumpers. I prefer the stainless-steel or chromed forms of both old-fashioned products.

In any case, hospitals and doctors have endorsed the bedpan with such enthusiasm that the instrument ought to take the place of the snakes-and-staff caduceus as a more fitting logo for the healing profession.

Several elegant investigations have proved conclusively that the average patient expends no more energy getting out of bed to use a commode than squiggling and worming onto a bedpan. And it's a heck of a lot easier psychologically and physiologically to go to the bathroom in a sitting position than when supine.

Despite the published studies that show no overall advantage to the bedpan, doctors still demand that patients use it. I believe the reason for this particular prejudice is rooted in some vague atavistic sadism that physicians desperately and unsuccessfully try to cover up. Perhaps our own toilet training was not all it should have been.

The bedpan has become a metaphor for hospital care: if it wasn't so unpleasant, everyone would want it. The bedpan is the primary reason so many sick people want to stay on their feet, in a manner of speaking. Obviously, the bedpan is the sole explanation for why our hospitals are not bursting with patients. The new Medicare rules pale into insignificance when compared to Bedpan Power as a force to keep people from demanding in-hospital care.

Any hospital that needs to double its census could do so almost overnight by banning bedpans. If nurses were relieved of bedpan duty, there would be raucous rejoicing by hordes of crisply starched RNs who would have so much unexpected leisure time on their hands that they would gratefully absorb the increasing amounts of menial paper work required of them. If the bedpan became a curiosity, doctors would want it back: we would claim that we were being deprived of our independence and freedom of choice. To physicians, the past is always more inspiring than the future; we worship the good old days.

Patient care would suffer (according to doctors) because of "government interference." Malpractice rates would skyrocket because opulent but chary insurance companies would claim increased risk of patients vaulting over the side rails to relieve themselves, and falling and breaking hips. No matter that this is a lie; the actuarial tables could prove anything.

The bedpan is the source of all medical woes. It could become the Cause of the Twentieth Century. We may properly excrete all our venom and frustration into (and take our resentments out on) the bedpan. This object of hate and defilement is designed to accept our emotional, as well as our physical, wastes. It serves no purpose other than to put a red ring on humanity's behind. I'll bet you can sense my growing intellectual momentum. Yes, hallelujah, brothers and sisters! What a revelation! The entire medical profession (now known familiarly as the mega-corporate-federal-health-maintenance-conglomerate) is ready to topple because it rests on . . . the bedpan.

THE INSIDE SCOOP

In 1974, a Senate report estimated that twelve thousand deaths a year resulted from surgery and prescription medicine. This figure was probably low in the 1970s, and it is undoubtedly an underestimation in the 1980s. According to a recent study, more than 35 percent of the patients in a university hospital suffered from unexpected "incidents." That estimate is probably also low, because it included only the unpleasant events that were reported. No one knows how many millions of patients experience iatrogenic (physician-caused) illnesses in offices and outpatient clinics, but the number must be astronomical.

One fact is clear: A hospital patient's risk of experiencing an untoward incident is high, and that risk increases proportionally the longer he or she is hospitalized.

Many physicians still take seriously the Hippocratic precept "Above all, do no harm." They are concerned about the risks inherent in modern technology and hospital care. There are, however, other doctors who readily accept iatrogenic illness as an unavoidable consequence of powerful drugs, difficult surgery and invasive medical testing. Unfortunately, these doctors are also apt to put up with sloppy care.

Hospitals claim they are concerned about errors and mistakes, but since hospitals are run by humans and humans have a tendency to err, there is little likelihood that you will get through an illness in a hospital, in this day and age, without a screw-up. There are just too many possibilities for things to go wrong in the average hospital for anyone to be able to control all of them. Doctors and nurses recognize this; that is why they will go to almost any length to avoid hospitalization.

Some years ago, when I saw George C. Scott in *The Hospital*, a movie billed as a comedy, I sat in the audience nodding my head in agreement while people around me screamed with laughter. To me, the scenes were not funny. They were true. As this brilliant satire unfolded, patients were killed off, one after another, by callousness, error and simple neglect.

If hospitals have mutated to the point where they can be dangerous, what can you say about them? Well, to begin with, they are wonderful places to visit if you want to find out the latest gossip. I wouldn't miss making daily rounds at the hospital, because in an hour or two I can find out exactly who's doing what to whom. Dr. Mergatroyd whispers dirty jokes and obscene proposals into the microphone when he dictates his discharge notes, but last week he was seen pinching the new dietary assistant. Does this mean he is no longer running after the evening operating room nurse? Will the anesthesiologist choose a new Hatteras yacht and be content to drive his Maserati for another year or two? Tune in tomorrow for the latest scoop.

The principles of hospital medical care are: Blood goes round and round; air goes in and out; oxygen is good. A handful of healers understand these fundamentals and act accordingly. A majority of physicians, however, believe in simpler principles, such as "I don't accept Medicare assignments" or "I can't take care of that because I am a specialist." It's been said that a well-trained physician knows what to do; an exceptionally well trained physician knows what not to do. As a rule, hospital doctors take the position that if you don't know what to do, do something.

Hospitals provide an effective way of treating depression. If a patient is depressed, it won't last long; he will cheer up when he sees how much worse off the other patients are. A hospital is not a place to be when you are so sick you can't get out of bed to summon a nurse. If you can stomach hospital food, you have no business being there. If you are lucky enough to be hospitalized for an incurable disease, take heart. Your chances of contracting a treatable illness are excellent. Then all the doctors and nurses can congratulate themselves on helping you get cured.

Of course, these comments are exaggerated. Hospitals are the pinnacle of American dedication to science. They soak up billions of health-care dollars for the purpose of buying expensive machines and training doctors who don't want to practice on their office patients. Hospitals are the last bastion of benevolence, altruism and charity. They are here to stay. But don't forget your insurance card the next time you go to one.

IS THAT TEST NECESSARY?

❖

You know you're a patient in a hospital when you hear the doctors in the corridor talking about "the Gallbladder in 803" or "the Coronary in 101," and you want to remind them that there's a human being surrounding the gallbladder (you). And if you're expected to subject yourself to multiple examinations by swarms of medical students, interns and residents, it's a good bet that you're a patient in a teaching or university hospital. (Excuse me, there are no more interns; somebody objected to the term "interns," so now we have "junior assistant residents," and they wear white coats just like the Big Guys.) Anyway, you have unending examinations—not for your sake, but for the sake of the young doctors whom you are helping to educate.

Okay, I buy that. It's the best way for physicians-in-training to learn, at the bedside. The process may be irritating for the patient, but it's inexpensive and accomplishes some good.

The next clue to your whereabouts in Sister Dolorosa Medical Center is the sudden realization that technicians are performing a lot of tests on you. These tests are sometimes dangerous; they are usually uncomfortable; they are always expensive. The situation prompted Dr. David Reuben, of Rhode Island Hospital in Providence, to write an article in the *New England Journal of Medicine*. What he said is not going to please residents . . . or interns.

To begin with, Dr. Reuben points out that "diagnostic evaluation has progressed beyond the capacities of therapeutic intervention." By this, he means that even if we have the power to substantiate a diagnosis, we are often helpless to cure the disease—or, for that matter, to alter its outcome.

Why, he asks, does the inexperienced doctor rely so heavily on testing? Because, he answers, physicians have a "desire to know." This desire is frequently translated into a caboodle of indiscriminate, unrelated laboratory investigations. This shotgun approach may help jittery residents to sleep better at night, he says, but "it should not be interpreted as constituting good medicine. In fact, it probably discourages analytic thinking and the development of good clinical judgment." There is, for instance, no valid justification for putting a person with end-stage heart disease through a gauntlet of further testing when common sense and decency tell us what is needed: warmth, concern, candor and whatever treatment may actually help.

In addition, testing runs up a big bill. One way or another, we all end up paying this bill, either directly or through increased insurance premiums. For example, the "desire to know" costs $55 million a year for the 225,000 patients with intestinal bleeding who undergo endoscopy. Such examinations are often just plain superfluous. If we are going to make a dent in the escalating costs of health care, we will have to begin insisting on diagnostic restraint. I am not suggesting that we suspend medical testing, but I believe we doctors have to be more discriminating. "If the outcome of a test will change therapy in a patient," says Dr. Reuben, "the physician should perform the safest test that will provide the necessary information to guide treatment."

Dr. Reuben acknowledges that any real change is unlikely

to come from within the academic institutions themselves. He exhorts practicing doctors and specialists "to forge a more sensible approach to diagnostic testing" by delineating the most appropriate tests, and then teaching students (and other doctors) to use them sparingly.

There was a time in medicine when clinical wisdom was a doctor's most valuable tool, his art and the key to good patient care. While no sane person would encourage a return to the guess-and-by-golly brand of prescientific healing, sound clinical judgment still has enormous application in today's medical world.

Part of being a doctor is having the ability to deal with ambiguity and uncertainty; often that's when physicians use their brains and skills to their fullest capacity. Professional healers must not equate the *ability* to know with the *need* to know. As Dr. Reuben notes: "The latter may at times be a luxury that may be neither beneficial nor affordable."

PATIENTS' RIGHTS: A VIEW FROM THE BED

❖

A nurse demands that you give up your medicine so that the hospital can supply the very same drugs you brought from home. Then she expects you to sign a consent for a special procedure, and the doctor hasn't explained what is going to take place. The night nurse officiously awakens you by shining a flashlight in your face to ask if you need a sleeping pill. Fictions? Not on your life. These are actual examples of what can happen to an unsuspecting patient who is admitted to a hospital.

Traditionally, when you become a hospital patient you are expected to abrogate many of the rights you enjoy and have come to expect as a healthy person. You tend to lose your identity and become a number, a nonthinking blob of protoplasm to be transported, poked, purged, bled, tested, serviced, occasionally

poisoned, often assaulted, and sometimes cut into. My colleagues may run me out of town on a rail, but it's my strong
feeling that a patient's vulnerability is a state of mind appreciated
by only a few of the personnel trained to care for the sick. If
you doubt what I say, I encourage you to become a hospital
patient from time to time. Fortunately, that option may not be
necessary much longer. More doctors, nurses and health professionals are becoming concerned about the unnecessary unpleasantness that can befall someone who is ill in the hospital.

To this end, a Patient's Bill of Rights was developed more
than ten years ago by the American Hospital Association. Although this document invariably makes hospital administrators
shudder, it deserves publicity because most hospitals have,
sometimes unbeknownst to their patients, adopted it or, at least,
agreed in theory with its tenets. I suppose the whole issue boils
down to humanism and caring. In general, small hospitals tend
to have fewer problems than do large hospitals. Please note that
I am not concerned, at the moment, with the quality of medical-
surgical care in hospitals. I am dealing only with the tendency
we all have to adopt stances that serve to magnify a patient's
loss of control. This can hardly be in the interests of the patient,
who is usually trying desperately to maintain control over his
own life, even in the face of illness. The Bill of Rights is worth
reviewing. In essence, it provides for the patient the right to:

1. Considerate and respectful care.
2. The name of the physician coordinating that care.
3. The names and functions of any allied personnel
   involved with that care.
4. Complete and current information about his diagnosis and treatment, given either to the patient or
   to the family, in understandable language.
5. Informed consent about any procedure or operation.
6. Refuse treatment to the extent permitted by law.
7. Reasonable privacy.
8. Confidentiality of all records.

9. A response by the hospital to reasonable demands by the patient for services.
10. Information about discharge plans and follow-up supervision.
11. Refuse to participate in research and experimentation.
12. Explanation of the hospital bill.
13. Know the hospital regulations that apply to his conduct as a patient.
14. Treatment without social or economic discrimination.

In essence, a sick person is still a person—whether or not he or she is hospitalized. Even those of us blessed with good health often need to be reminded of that fact; we never know when we, too, may need hospitalization.

BE A BETTER HOSPITAL VISITOR

❖

With today's confusing and complex hospital life, patients are often baffled by routines that may seem natural and simple to the hospital staff. Likewise, visitors may not feel comfortable because they are not sure how to react to hospital regulations or to people who are ill. Here are ten rules to help visitors become better attuned to patients' needs.

1. Don't bring food or medicine to patients unless you have received prior approval to do so. I have been involved in several situations in which well-wishers brought in food, cigarettes and even alcoholic beverages to sick patients. While you may be eager to make a patient's hospital stay as "normal" as possible, such largess can often undo therapy and actually prolong a patient's

hospitalization. Please don't be an unsanctioned Santa. You may be doing more harm than good.

2. Do not bring your personal problems or business decisions into the hospital room. The sick person is often having enough trouble dealing with being vulnerable and dependent and doesn't need the added burden of extraneous worries. Although this rule may seem self-evident, I am aware of an instance in which a visitor sneaked into an intensive care unit to ask a postoperative patient when the visitor's lawn mower would be fixed. Please do not add unnecessarily to a patient's stress.

3. Be sensitive to patients' needs. Don't interrupt meals, arrive at bathtime, hover in the room when personnel are carrying out vital functions or examinations. If you have to be asked to leave, you shouldn't have been there in the first place.

4. Don't argue with the staff. Nurses and paramedical employees are trained to administer fundamentals of treatment that, in general, are designed for the benefit of the patient. Although hospitals are often impersonal and sometimes frustrating places, the staff is professional. If you have a complaint, don't make a scene in the patient's presence. Rather, review the issue with the doctor or nurse in charge—out of the patient's earshot. Vociferous arguments do not help the healing process, especially when the confrontation occurs at the bedside.

5. Time your visit so as not to overlap with other callers. Most hospitals limit the number of persons who can simultaneously see a patient. This rule has a sound basis. Visitors are tiring; in a sense, they have to be "entertained." Patients are not up to this social commitment. Two or three visitors at a time are about the limit a bed patient can tolerate. In addition, even if the patient you are visiting can enjoy the company, the constant influx of "guests" into a semiprivate room can be exhausting to the other patients in the room. Privacy is hard to come by in a hospital; hordes of visitors make privacy an impossibility. Check with the family or the nurse to establish an appropriate schedule. Please don't think it amusing to cram several people into a patient's room. Even though you may have been successful in

bypassing the front desk and the nurses' station (and believe yourself to be one degree below James Bond for breaching hospital security), this insensitive behavior can have an adverse effect on the patient's recovery. One more observation: Most hospitals are willing to "bend the rules"—in particular with respect to young children and out-of-town family visitors. Please get permission before you take it upon yourself to visit with youngsters or at odd times.

6. Don't be noisy or boisterous. Sound travels in hospitals. Furthermore, hospital rooms are small. Although I am not urging you to behave like the proverbial church mouse, I am suggesting that the decibel level be reasonable. We already have a problem with noise from hospital staff. Hospitals are working to reduce this. The additional racket made by unthinking visitors compounds the stress on patients, particularly during the evening hours. Try to be reserved and considerate.

7. Be natural in your approach to a patient. By this I mean that neither optimism nor unnecessary discouragement have a place in the patient's room. Patients wish to be told the truth, but that truth can be told in a manner that will facilitate recovery—or at least minimize anguish. Most patients are involved in a therapeutic program that can be severely undermined by unthinking visitors who are not acting in conjunction with the family or the doctor.

8. Don't smoke in a patient's room. I will not reiterate the malignant effects of tobacco smoke. For the patient—even a smoker—who is recuperating, smoke always exerts a disagreeable effect. Patients are not helped by inhaling the smoke from visitors' cigarettes, pipes or cigars. The request that visitors not smoke is so basic that it's hard to believe it still needs mentioning. Yet, time and again, I see visitors smoking in hospital rooms. Don't do it. If you cannot last an hour without tobacco, you yourself ought to be a patient—or may well be in the future.

9. When you visit, pick a time that is consistent with hospital regulations. Again, there are reasons for this limitation. Patients must bathe, eat, undergo treatments and examinations. Receiv-

ing company at these rather personal times can be disruptive to hospital routine and to patients' privacy. Although hospitals are sometimes willing to adjust these rules, please obtain prior permission for such exceptions.

10. Don't stay too long. Patients tire easily, particularly those who are seriously ill or in pain. Often they are embarrassed to ask visitors to leave for fear of hurting their feelings. Be perceptive. If there are nonverbal messages being broadcast by the patient, please heed them. In short, try to empathize with the patient—and act accordingly.

For the most part, visitors are thoughtful, well-motivated, caring persons who wish to give what support they can in uncomfortable situations. Although all callers may attempt to be "good" visitors, perhaps—with some reflection—there is room for improvement.

Don't forget that being sick is no fun; it is terrifyingly disruptive. Please be considerate, and if you have questions or complaints, leave the bedside and resolve them with the appropriate authority. The charge nurse, in particular, is a valuable asset. She (or he) can help familiarize you with hospital policy and ways in which you may contribute to the patient's recovery.

A HARD WAY TO MAKE A LIVING

❖

In the hospital to which I admit patients, there are signs that proclaim: "If you think nurses are second-class citizens, try running a first-class hospital without them." These signs are correct. Nurses are vital resources. At the same time, they are misunderstood, exploited, depreciated and underpaid.

I hear people say that nurses are no longer dedicated to their profession. Such a fallacious statement is not worthy of comment. Any person privileged to work with nurses cannot help but be impressed with the dedication they show.

To begin with, nurses assume responsibilities that would have been unthinkable a few years ago. In addition to their traditional duties of making patients more comfortable—a full-time job in its own right—they are now called upon to dispense powerful drugs on delicate schedules, deal with vast record keeping and paper work, function in high-pressure situations and continue to maintain close personal contact with (and a supportive environment for) sick people.

You may be surprised to learn that nursing is an extremely physical occupation. Watch a good hundred-pound nurse perform all necessary services for a belligerent and confused two-hundred-pound postoperative patient; you will begin to understand what true exertion is and how principles of leverage can be used to their greatest advantage.

It's a hell of a way to make a living. Doctors characteristically view nurses as handmaidens or, in the case of male nurses, valets. In addition to caring for the sick and the vulnerable, nurses have to deal with doctors who, unfortunately, are often as demanding as the patients. A mistake in ordering medicine may be translated into an error of administration; the nurse takes the guff for what is really the physician's responsibility. Because the doctors' authority is perceived as beyond question, they often berate—yes, actually yell at—nurses who have the temerity to question what they are doing.

Finally, nurses' salaries are abominable. Fully employed registered nurses earn an average of $18,000 yearly (with a range of $13,000 to $25,000). They work forty-hour weeks, including nights and weekends. The highest salaries go to nurses working in administrative positions. The average earnings of a hospital general nurse are about $16,000, or $8 an hour.

To compound the problem, "vertical mobility" (the chance for advancement) is almost nonexistent in the profession. A head nurse may earn $9 an hour, or slightly more, depending upon what part of the country she chooses to work in. For example, staff nurses in small New England hospitals earn far less than psychiatric nurses in large, federally funded hospitals in the far west. The salary difference between a floor nurse and a director of nursing can be as little as $6.00 versus $9.65 an hour. And once a nurse, because of seniority or skill, reaches the top of the ladder for her area, she cannot expect additional salary increases. By all criteria, nurses are underpaid.

We are experiencing changes in the field of nursing care: more male nurses, flexibility in dress, increased responsibility, more nonnurses performing mundane but essential services, specialization, accentuated militancy of R.N.s' justified demands for recognition. These changes are necessary for a healthy, vibrant profession.

Nurses deserve our understanding and support. Theirs is a fine and honorable profession. It's time their first-class status was reaffirmed. To do less is to undermine the exceptionally high level of health care we are privileged to enjoy in this country.

BRAVO!

❖

There are few more potentially rewarding and pleasurable medical disciplines than the acute care of the premature infant. I am certain that saving young lives constitutes a continuing miracle for doctors who have chosen the super specialty of neonatology.

I know from a parent's viewpoint that nothing can compare to the wonder of watching a "preemie" survive and develop. I know because, as a parent, I was there. I held my breath under the fluorescent lights in the hectic but strangely subdued, climate-controlled nursery. Among the chromed pumps and huffing respiratory machines, the jungle vines of intravenous tubing and chalk-white feeding lines, I helplessly marveled at modern technology and dedication.

Our premature daughter died several years ago in a newborn care unit. Benjamin, who weighed two pounds at birth and spent his first three months of life in the same unit, recently celebrated his seventh birthday. He made it.

Several years ago, the Newborn Special Care Unit at Yale– New Haven Medical Center celebrated its twentieth birthday. The event was commemorated at a gigantic picnic near the Yale Bowl. Parents, staff and alumni were invited to rejoice in improved newborn survival, a happy new phenomenon. In all fairness, I should emphasize that most large teaching hospitals sustain units specifically designed and operated for the treatment of sick newborns and premature infants. All these units are accomplishing medical magic, making astonishing advances that have become almost commonplace in the past twenty years. Hyaline membrane disease is no longer always fatal. Antibiotics have reduced the incidence of epidemic infections in nurseries. There is more awareness and avoidance of drugs (including alcohol and tobacco), which, when used by mothers-to-be, can result in fetal abnormalities. Brilliantly delicate operations now can be performed upon even the youngest baby in order to correct life-threatening congenital abnormalities. Smaller infants are surviving; the 70 percent mortality in neonates weighing less than a kilogram (2.2 pounds) has been reduced to 18 percent. And desperately tiny newborns are being saved. Newborns weighing as little as one and a half pounds can survive if they are treated in special nurseries. Finally, factors causing brain damage in infants of any birth weight are being mastered.

Neonatologists concede that many problems are yet to be solved. Malnutrition, teen-age pregnancy (far more devastating and dangerous than maternity in older women), premature labor and genetic defects remain catastrophic issues for both parents and their children.

Still, it is comforting to know that phenomenal efforts are being made, on a twenty-four-hour basis, by thousands of talented, devoted—and often exhausted—doctors, nurses, technicians and volunteers. Their unpublicized goal is to permit another tiny, wrinkled, dependent, unappreciative packet of energy to live and grow. We all—parents and nonparents—owe these hospital professionals an incalculable debt.

CHAPTER 6

WHY DOES IT COST SO MUCH?

DIALING FOR DOCTORS

❖

Doctors' receptionists are vital. They can make or break a practice. And, as you may see from the following one-sided telephone conversation, they have been superbly instructed by their employers.

"Good morning. Dr. Mergatroyd's office. ... I said, Dr. Mergatroyd's office. ... Hello? Oh, there you are.

"No, he's not in. You want an appointment? Is this for a complete exam or just an office visit?

"Well, for all new patients, the doctor insists on a cardiogram, chest X ray, sigmoid exam and blood tests. ...

"About three hundred and seventy-five dollars. Hello? An office visit then. What's the problem?

"No one gets colds anymore. You must have the flu. The doctor will surely want a chest X ray and...

"That's impossible. The doctor doesn't make house calls.

"All right. He can see you next Thursday at four. ... What do you mean you could be dead by then? Look, I'm very busy. ...

"Just a slight fever and hacky cough? That's all? Very well. I'll make an exception. Come Tuesday at three.

"What? How much for an office visit? Well, it depends. Ordinarily, it's fifty dollars for the first visit.

"Yes, for just a cold ... I mean the flu.

"I'm sorry you feel that way. Do you want an appointment or not?

"Tuesday at three then. Oh, I should remind you. The doctor doesn't accept Medicare. ... That's right. You'll be expected to pay at the time of your visit.

"... Or check, whichever you prefer. Also, there is a five-dollar malpractice surcharge. Yes, it's something new. The doctor's rates went way up. Excuse me a minute. ... [to patient in office] I know you've been waiting for an hour. Dr. Mergatroyd is very busy. You'll just have to be patient. I don't know where he is. Now please sit down—I'm busy on the phone....

"Hello? Yes, I'm back. I want to remind you to be prompt. If you cancel your appointment less than twenty-four, hours in advance, there will be a no-show charge...

"Yes, you heard me—a no-show charge of twenty dollars....

"No, it's not ridiculous. The doctor's time is precious.

"I know you plan to be here. I'm just trying to inform you about how our office operates.

"Oh, one other thing. You'll have to fill out your own insurance forms, so bring them with you. . . . What? *Of course* I'll lend you a pen.

"All right. Tuesday at three. What's your name?

"Never married, eh? What was the problem? . . . Well, never mind. Where do you live? . . . Mmm, not a very good neighborhood, is it? On second thought, you'd better bring cash. The doctor has had people bounce checks before.

"You'd better figure at least seventy-five dollars for a ten-minute visit and tests....

"I told you already. A chest X ray and maybe a blood count. If you run over the allotted time, there's a small additional charge of two dollars per minute....

"You needn't be nasty. . . . Of course it's a business—the business of curing the sick. . . . Yes, that's right, curing the sick....

"He has to eat too, you know, just like the rest of us.

"We all live on fixed incomes, honey. Look, I really don't have time to argue. Hello? Hello?

"Can you believe that? She hung up!"

BUCK-PASSERS WHO PASS YOUR BUCKS

❖

Of all the defense mechanisms used by the average human being to avoid responsibility, one has worked so well for doctors that it is now as much a part of medical practice as are tax shelters and computer billing. This mechanism is called denial, and doctors are the quintessential proponents of it.

Take medical expenses, for example. Although most physicians acknowledge that medical care is becoming financially exorbitant, few doctors are willing to admit that the good old practitioner is a major cause of escalating costs. The real causes, they say, are hospitals and the "new technology" demanded by patients. This misperception is almost universal among doctors, because it removes responsibility from the physician and places it on Them—uncaring hospital administrators and the eternally unsatisfied public.

But wait. Who decides when patients should enter hospitals and how long they should stay? Who orders astronomical constellations of X rays and lab tests? Who determines which treatments are used? Who charges you $1,500 for an operation and then hits you up for fifty bucks every time he sticks his head in the door of your hospital room to say hello? Your doctor, folks.

To make matters worse, physicians rarely know the costs of the services and drugs that are ordered. Incredibly, we don't even care. An M.D. who speculates heavily in buffalo-hide futures can rattle off three weeks of high–low figures. He knows the cost of a new Maserati Biturbo without even thinking. The amount he socked away in his Keogh and yesterday's closing price of his computer stock are irrevocably programmed into his brain. But he can't for the life of him remember how much a blood chem-screen costs, although he orders them every day for his patients.

I am not familiar with any doctors who know what their associates charge. On second thought, maybe some surgeons are privy to this privileged information. However, the average physician would no more ask another doctor what he charges for an office examination than he would inquire how much Scotch the old boy puts away after hours. If you really want to make a doctor suffer, ask him precisely what the hospital radiologist is paid for reading an abdominal ultrasound exam or how much the anesthesiologist will stick you for a spinal. You might get a figure if you ask what your doctor himself charges for an office call, but you'll be put in a class with E.T. if you demand that he tell you what his surgical colleagues make from hernia operations.

As an ordinary consumer, you price things when you shop. You're entitled to an estimate before you agree to have a valve job on your car. When you buy heating oil, you know what the stuff costs per gallon before it's delivered. When you buy a sports coat or a dress, the price is on the sleeve. In short, you're able to plan ahead and know the extent of your commitment.

However, in a hospital it's all very vague, mystical and unspoken. There are hidden charges too—everything from Band-Aids to blood-drawing fees—that can show up weeks later on your bill.

If you want to feel the hair rise on your neck, read a hospital bill. Doctors occasionally read them and are astounded, but we soon forget. We deny. It's all for the good of the patient, you know. And the doctor doesn't want to give up the right to spend your money as he sees fit. We want to stay in control. We insist that you do what we think is best for you. So it becomes the fault of the hospital—or the moon or Japanese imports—that charges are high. Forget that the doctor was responsible for them in the first place. We are experts at passing the buck—literally.

I've conceived of a method to fix all this. First, every patient needs an itemized bill. More important, the fees for separate services ought to be listed on all lab requisitions so that doctors are constantly reminded how much each test costs. Finally, a patient should be entitled to the doctor's preadmission estimate of hospital expense in a nonemergency.

Of course, the medical establishment would scream bloody murder. Then, while they're having conniption fits, ask the doctors to pay a portion of the charges over and above the estimate. Crash. Bang. Boom.

Hey! C'mon, guys, take it easy; I'm only kidding.

LET THE HILTON HANDLE HERNIAS

According to an article in *The New York Times* not long ago, the Mount Sinai Medical Center in Manhattan has been granted permission by state health planners to spend almost $500 million to upgrade its medical complex. The hospital will tear down ten of its twenty-six buildings, add a new 633-bed wing, renovate its private pavilions, build new operating rooms, enlarge its emergency suite and generally tidy things up a bit.

If you were to become a patient in the institution after the project's completion, you would be asked to pay a base rate of $569 for each night spent in the hospital. This figure is for room and board only; it does not include doctors' fees and the scores of additional charges tacked on the bill by the hospital.

As part of the compromise needed to gain state approval, Mount Sinai agreed to join the city's 911 emergency system and "to help improve the quality of medical care for the people in predominantly black and Hispanic East Harlem."

I don't know how many of you have been hospitalized recently in a prestigious center like Mount Sinai, but I can tell you it's no vacation. The food isn't four-star. Drinks are not on the house. There are no double beds. The staff—probably extremely competent—is not, however, geared up to anticipate your every need and grant your every wish. You do not get to sleep soundly at night because that's when the interns do their thing and night nurses can't stand a nestful of quietly slumbering patients. These damsels are young and want a little action on the eleven-to-seven shift. They want some rowdiness, a little fun and noise—anything to keep the interns awake and interested.

In short, a hospital is not the kind of place you go to for a rest . . . especially if you are not feeling up to par.

Off the top of my head, I can think of several resorts where you could have a whale of a good time for $569 a night. I've never been to these spots, but I'll wager you could have a real blowout. Also, getting there is half the fun, unlike picking your way over the garbage and avoiding a mugging between 98th and 102nd streets, where Mount Sinai nestles.

I wouldn't be surprised to learn that five hundred bucks would get you a nice suite at one of New York's better hotels—complete with free parking, room service and a French maid. Maybe even a good floor show. And your spouse, or current nearest-and-dearest, could accompany you to share in the festivities.

I think hospitals are vying with hotels for the tourist trade. But it's just a flash in the pan.

Hotels don't have a chance as long as Medicare and medical insurance pick up the tab. Have you ever heard of an employer offering vacation insurance? Something like $800 a day, if you're disabled, for two weeks in Acapulco? No, hospitals have the edge, and they know it. You're willing to put up with food that's been steam-wilted, interns who are surly and bleary-eyed, nurses who stick an amazing array of objects into your every orifice, because . . . because you're kinky? Not on your life. Because it's free! It's a health lottery, and you, neighbor, have just won the grand prize: a glorious ten-day getaway to Municipal Hospital! Retail value, $5,690. Tips not included. Void where prohibited by law.

Some of you may truly believe that hospitals are nonprofit, humane organizations whose reason for existence is to serve the sick and make them well. I won't argue the point. But if that's true, how come *Business Week* reported that David A. Jones, chairman of Humana, Inc.—the third-largest hospital holding company, with eighty-six acute-care hospitals—earned $18,116,000 in 1984? Does he know something we don't?

I have a suggestion for a budding entrepreneur. If a nationally known hotel chain could be enticed to offer free X rays, blood tests and hernia operations, and if we could convince an insurance company to issue special policies...

THE MEGA-ECONOMICS OF A SURGEON

❖

The task of bringing health expenses into line is viewed by most people as something like balancing a paper clip on end; sure, it can be done as a trick, but as a normal state of affairs, no way.

Although I have no objection to reasonable surgical fees—I believe these specialists have every right to fair compensation—I am periodically astounded to learn what some surgeons demand and receive as recompense for a few hours' work. For example, cardiovascular surgeons are amply paid for what they do: $8,000 to $10,000 for each coronary-artery bypass procedure are the usual figures that are bandied about. That seems like a lot of money to me, and I have developed the unpleasant habit of badgering these surgeons about their fees.

A few months ago, I had the privilege of participating in a surprisingly frank discussion with a heart surgeon. This extremely qualified expert was, in the 1960s, a pioneer of the coronary bypass procedure. He went on to become chairman of several departments of heart surgery in some of New York City's most prestigious teaching hospitals. He subsequently discontinued active surgery because life "in the fast lane" was not for him and, I suspect, he became disillusioned with the mega-economics of heart surgery. For reasons of confidentiality, I will not mention him by name. I've modified the precise wording of the following exchange; the sentiments and facts, however, are fairly represented.

"So you were one of the first surgeons to perform coronary bypass?" I asked.

"Yes," he replied. "When I started, the operation was largely experimental. Only a handful of surgeons were performing the procedure."

"How did you decide how much to charge?"

"Well," he answered, "none of us knew what a fair charge would be. I hadn't any experience with the money side of the thing, so I went and talked to an older surgeon who was then the department chairman. He told me to put in for an astronomical figure—I think it was three thousand or four thousand dollars—and then see what the insurance companies thought."

"That was a lot of money in those days," I volunteered, remembering that I was charging $3 for an office call in the 1960s. "What sort of reaction did you expect?"

"It's funny," he mused. "We really believed we would be turned down flat, or at least they'd substantially reduce our proposal. But they didn't. They accepted it without blinking an eye."

"The whole four thousand dollars?"

"Yes. No questions asked. We started operating as soon as we could, and there was no problem with reimbursement. Since then, the fee has continued to rise, of course. I think I was getting about eight thousand dollars a procedure when I quit, and I was doing three cases a day."

"Let's see," I mumbled, "that's a hundred and twenty thousand for a five-day week, fifty weeks a year. Not bad: six million dollars a year."

"Yeah, something in that range."

"Why do you suppose the insurance companies accepted the original figure?"

He paused and rubbed his chin. "I think they were eager to keep the price high so that patients would be convinced that health insurance was necessary. They wanted to sell insurance policies. They hungered for those premiums. They wanted to be indispensable to the public."

I hope this conversation is as informative for you as it was for me. The surgeon's observations truly put certain medical costs in a different light, don't they?

SALT ON THE STREETS— AND ON THE WOUNDS

On the basis of a study performed for the Health Care Financing Administration, scientists concluded that about 25 percent of hospital admissions are unjustified, and that up to 50 percent of laboratory tests may be unwarranted.

Small wonder that billions of health dollars are wasted every year.

A survey of twenty-four Iowa hospitals revealed that by age fifteen, 70 percent of children in one section of the state had tonsillectomies; only 7 percent in another area had the operation. A portion of New Hampshire is blessed with six times more hospital admissions for tooth extractions than a similar community in nearby Vermont. Uncomplicated obstetrical attention in northeast area hospitals results in 50 percent longer stays than in corresponding institutions in western states.

In one part of the country, physicians who order myriad laboratory tests are considered to be "tinkering"; in another region, they may be viewed as simply "thorough." The cost of medical care varies extensively among different communities; it even varies from one hospital to another within these communities.

This crisis of consistency has reached such proportions that the National Blue Cross and Blue Shield Association has issued guidelines that define under what circumstances certain medical tests are reimbursable by member insurance companies. Blue

Cross–Blue Shield is trying like the dickens to reduce redundancy. For example, if you have a breast lump, there is no economically justifiable reason for the doctor to order a bevy of investigations—like sonography, mammography, thermography and diaphanography—when one or, at most, two tests will suffice.

Pretty soon, the Blues aren't going to pay for laboratory analyses whose purposes are questionable. It is only a matter of time before "guidelines" become translated into dollars-and-cents reality. The meat-ax approach to trimming medical expenses will necessitate that each patient and doctor work toward the most frugal methods of establishing diagnosis.

Physicians become righteously indignant when economists mess around with the marketplace and with doctors' God-given right to run the show. I understand this indignation, but understanding is not going to make the problem go away.

Most doctors order too many tests, and that is a simple fact of medical life. For years, we, as a profession, have abused our patients' pocketbooks. Since we still oversee and control the health industry, we have an obligation to address the issue of medical costs before the responsibility is taken from us.

Learning to exercise good judgment in the administration of medical care is superior to the option of depriving some Americans of health care because they can't afford it. Patients have to be educated to want, and practitioners to deliver, more cost-effective care. The question is: How?

In my part of the country, highway-maintenance crews spend all night plowing winter roads that are barely dusted with snow. Another favorite trick is salting bare streets. It's all too much. My rocker panels last about two years. I sometimes think that the state's department of transportation actively subsidizes body shops. In winter, the avenues and thoroughfares are slushy examples of chemical zealotry, saline testimonials to "bare at any cost," dripping reminders that Nature can be beaten back at time-and-a-half overtime.

I'm certain that formal complaints by the public enjoy the same fate as irate letters from patients about exorbitant bills for anesthesia and surgery. Nothing gets done; the system is so enormous that it continues on its trajectory without even a wobble. I hate to say it, but you have about as much control over road salt and medical costs as you do over the weather next St. Patrick's Day.

Until Medicare and private insurance companies cooperate in a nationwide effort to reduce profligate spending, medical costs will continue to rise, while each of us complains about corpulent taxes and bloated insurance premiums.

Meanwhile, don't forget to hose off the undercarriage of your vehicle periodically... or in about five years, you'll be lucky to be able to sell it for scrap.

GLADYS AND ESTHER: A TALE OF THE EMERGENCY ROOM

❖

DEAR GLADYS,

Greetings from the sunny southland! I saw on the hotel TV that you had ten inches of snow last Tuesday and nothing was moving in the city. Sure made me glad Herb and I came south this year. His emphysema has really been acting up since he retired. He just can't take the cold anymore.

I hope you got the grapefruit we sent. The oranges didn't look so good this year, and they were pretty expensive too.

Listen, I've got to tell you what happened last week. Herb and I were in the shopping mall and it was hot and I hadn't had much breakfast—you know, just a Danish and some coffee—and I sort of slipped coming out of a boutique. Maybe I got a little dizzy or something. You know how I am in the morning. Anyway, down I went. I didn't really get hurt, but I twisted my ankle and couldn't stand on it.

Well, you would of thought I was the Pope or that star Fara What's-her-name. The store manager called an ambulance, and before you could say "Trapper John," I was in the hospital emergency room. Gladys, you wouldn't believe the scene! It was just like on TV with all those cute young doctors in funny blue uniforms. The doctors were so young! I haven't been to an E.R. (see? I even picked up the medical lingo!) since Herb had asthma from the flu in '82.

I had to wait a long time to be seen because a lot of people there had colds, rashes and sore throats. But finally this really sweet assistant resident (I think he called himself)—just a kid, really, no older than my grandson—this resident took me into an examining room. He called me Esther, so friendly like, and introduced himself as Dr. Wicks. Then he asked me what happened, and I explained that my ankle hurt because I twisted it. He took a quick look and said I would need X rays, blood tests and maybe something called a bone scan. All for a little sprain? I couldn't believe it. When I was a little girl, old Doc Williams would poke around, pat your behind, tell you to come back tomorrow if it hurt, and send you out to play. What a difference now! This must be what they call "technology." I said to this nice young Dr. Wicks, "Aren't those tests expensive? Who's going to pay?" He was very reassuring and said not to worry. Medicare would pay some and the store owner had insurance, so what difference did the expense make? Esther, he said, you're the kind of person who should go first-class.

You know, Gladys, I realized then and there that all this talk about high medical costs is really about other people, not about me. Dr. Wicks said that when it comes to you yourself, cost is not the object and the doctor wants you to have the best, sort of like the senators and big shots who get free care at Walter Reed, I think it is. Dr. Wicks said, "Leave it to me, honey." Wasn't that sweet? Honestly, Gladys, that resident was so cute.

So, anyway, I had all the tests he ordered. Everything was normal and I didn't need the bone scan because—lucky me— the X rays were normal. After about three hours, the nurse wrapped my ankle with an Ace bandage. She gave me crutches and an instruction sheet and sent me back to the hotel. Of course, the day was spoiled, but I sure had an education sitting in that

E.R. watching all the people. It was even more interesting than watching *General Hospital*, and there were no commercials.

I tell you, hospitals are the way to go. Everybody's so busy and so—I don't know—competent is the best word, I guess. None of our friends down here can even get into a doctor's office without having a complete checkup and tests, tests, tests! Believe me, that's expensive. Herb's friend Larry had to have a cardiogram and blood sugar test just for a little ingrown toenail. He finally went to a foot doctor—no M.D., you can bet—and got fixed up in two days. No wonder all the people with minor ailments come to the E.R. where insurance pays for everything and you don't have to wait three weeks for an appointment. If that's socialized medicine, I'm all for it.

Gladys, I must confess I really missed not being able to talk more to Dr. Wicks. He was in such a hurry that everything was one-sided. *He* did all the talking. It was slam, bam, thank you, ma'am. Much too rushed for an old lady like me. He didn't seem to care too much about the ankle and kept mumbling words like "liability" under his breath. I wish he had taken more time to examine my foot and less time fiddling around with all those tests. He didn't even bother to ask me about my arthritis.

Well, Herb just got back from golf, so I'll say goodbye for now. We'll be home in about a week. Please don't forget to give the super the twenty dollars we left him. Say hi to the Murphys.

Affectionately,

ESTHER

CHAPTER 7

AN
INFORMED
CONSUMER
MAKES
THE BEST
PATIENT

❖

GREAT EXPECTATIONS

❖

The medical profession seems to many people to be a cornucopia: medicine and its allied professions appear to have the capacity to solve any health problem. In particular, there must be a drug for any illness. Part of the problem, I suppose, has to do with expectations. Today's patients expect to get well if they seek help. When they do not get well, they become angry and blame the doctor, the hospital or the government. Or they sue everyone in sight.

Of course, medical science does not have all the answers. Doctors are not all-knowing; our fund of knowledge is pitifully small. Yet I share the public's unrealistic expectations. I am caught up in the same sort of optimistic enthusiasm. And I too become angry at bad results, incensed at unsolved problems, critical of deficiencies. My bloated expectations probably stem from one of the great revolutions of this country: the development of healing drugs and chemicals.

Twenty years ago, high blood pressure was a serious and often disabling illness—primarily because treatment was unsatisfactory. We used two basic drugs: diuretics and reserpine. The diuretics produced enhanced urine formation, thereby ridding the hypertensive of unwanted extra water. Most diuretics were of the thiazide class and there were side effects—diabetes, depletion of body minerals (especially potassium), gout, nausea, vomiting, rash, jaundice and other unsavory conditions. Reserpine was a relatively pure form of *Rauwolfia serpentina* and, as such, caused severe mental changes, particularly depression and suicidal tendencies. Dangerous? You bet. But, except for some experimental drugs, they were all we had.

In the 1960s other medications became available. Although

physicians would still begin treatment with diuretics, there were highly effective "secondary" or "backup" medicines. All had substantial side effects ranging from impotence to life-threatening anemia.

During the past few years, still another class of drugs—the beta blockers—has been developed. They hold great promise; side effects are less severe and easier to control. As hypertension becomes better understood, new drugs can be utilized to achieve desired goals.

Hypertension is now known to be caused in many cases by an excess quantity of a certain chemical named angiotensin II. A new drug, now widely available, specifically blocks the formation of angiotensin II. If the experts are correct, we may be on the threshold of successfully and selectively treating high blood pressure without the use of diuretics or any secondary medication.

It's hard to avoid being enthusiastic about the possibility of taming one of man's common diseases. Before becoming too smug, we had best remind ourselves that many other diseases— notably heart disease and cancer—remain scourges in the purest medieval sense.

We still have a long way to go. If we can manage to keep our expectations under control, who knows what next year will bring? Please be kind to scientists and health professionals. They see the chasm between what is needed and what is available. They know that no profession has the capability to solve all the problems we share. An informed and patient public with realistic expectations is a vital factor in the successful use of medications.

GENERIC VERSUS BRAND-NAME DRUGS

Most medicines are complex, relatively sophisticated compounds. Although they may be difficult to manufacture, the real challenge comes in the purification process, when the active ingredients are extracted. To use a simple analogy, a good cook can make excellent vegetable soup from scratch. However, think of the job he or she would have extracting from the pot only that portion containing celery and celery water. Such a task could not be carried out in a kitchen, nor would any sane cook wish to repeat the process over and over.

In many ways, a similar chore confronts drug manufacturers. A purified medicine must be separated from the chemical brew in which it is "cooked." The methods of performing this feat are complicated and must be carried out with exquisite precision, batch after batch, year after year. It's an expensive proposition.

Also, the techniques and final products must constantly be analyzed to ensure purity. Doctors do not wish to prescribe (nor do patients wish to purchase) drugs that are sloppily made and may contain contaminants. Aspirin, as medicine goes, is easy to make. One of our projects in college organic chemistry was to make aspirin in the laboratory, and if a bunch of scruffy twenty-year-old students can make it, anybody can. Of course, our product was so impure it wasn't fit for sick pigs. Nonetheless, we learned that the manufacturing process was no piece of cake.

In any case, purity and reliability are crucial for pharmaceutical companies. This brings me to my point: generic versus brand-name medicine.

When a drug manufacturer markets a compound, the medication is renamed. There are many reasons for this. One is that chemicals have long names that do not lend themselves to retailing. Consumers are much less inclined to order, and doctors to remember, the generic trihexyphenidyl than its brand name, Artane—the anti-Parkinson's disease product by Lederle.

In addition, by promising purity and uniformity, the manufacturer hopes its brand will become synonymous with quality and will, therefore, be prescribed to the exclusion of lower-grade generics. For example, Lederle once captured a large portion of the tetracycline market because its brand, Achromycin, contained what it was supposed to contain: exactly 250 mg. of purified tetracycline per blue-and-yellow capsule.

Some years ago, a study revealed that the heart pill digoxin had enormous variability in potency and strength, depending on where it was made. Only Lanoxin, by Burroughs Wellcome, was consistent, and it became the gold standard for digoxin preparations.

Although pharmaceutical profits are quite acceptable—particularly if a company hits a real winner like Valium (diazepam by Roche) or Tagamet (cimetidine by Smith Kline and French)—it costs a lot of money to run a first-class quality-control program. One way to cut overhead is to manufacture medicine cheaply and reduce quality control. This is precisely what is being done by many less sophisticated drug companies, especially those in other countries.

Patients and doctors are often unaware that the generic version may not be up to snuff. A decade or so ago, tetracycline made in Italy and sold in this country was found to vary all over the place in purity and potency. In a study released in 1980, scientists reported that brand-name manufacturers were responsible for 70 percent of all drug production, but were subject to less than 20 percent of all drug recalls.

The brand-name-versus-generic dilemma is very much a problem in today's medical world. We all want quality at reasonable prices. However, as one alert physician from Indiana reminded me, we tend to disregard the fact that there is much more cost variation among pharmacies than there is between brand-name drugs and their generic equivalents. Consumers usually will get a better deal by price shopping than by insisting on generic brands only. Patients will always obtain a more satisfactory product by purchasing drugs manufactured by a trustworthy pharmaceutical house, whether those drugs are brand-name or generic. The brand-name brouhaha is based less on the names of medicines than it is on the issue of who makes them.

To make sure you are getting what you need, you may have to lean heavily on your pharmacist. Don't accept medicine made by companies whose dependability and reliability have not been proved. If you do, you may be getting less (or more, or something different) than you bargained for.

FEAR
OF
FRYING

❖

Patients have the right to honest answers about radiation. All of us are constantly bombarded by X rays from our environment—sun, stones, soil—so-called background radiation. We have little control over the presence of unstable atoms in nature, and, fortunately for most of us, the amount is small. But we can control contact with man-made radiation, and judging from the facts, that control is overdue.

The average American absorbs yearly about 180 millirems: 75 percent comes from natural sources, the remainder from medical and dental X rays. Years ago, experts believed that low-level radiation (less than 1,000 millirems a year) was safe. In the past twenty years, many studies have disproved this view. Now all official regulatory agencies class *any* radiation as potentially harmful. That is, even low-level amounts can affect health.

For example, an unborn child exposed to 300 to 800 millirems from its mother's pelvic X ray is statistically more likely to develop any of a variety of childhood cancers. Older patients, who had frequent fluoroscopy for lung disease, have a four-to-eightfold increase in breast cancer. Often, such unfortunate consequences take many years to develop.

All radiation causes cell disruption at the molecular level, where DNA—the stuff that determines a cell's formation—can be altered and permanently changed. Obviously, any method we can use to minimize X-ray exposure will, in the long run, be beneficial.

For obvious reasons, doctors tend to underplay the amount of radiation in diagnostic tests. Therefore, you may be unpleasantly surprised to read the following chart, which I have adapted from *Consultant* (January 1984). Radiation doses are expressed in millirems.

Type of Study	Total Body Dose	Bone-Marrow Dose	Gonad Dose
dental bite	5	1	0
dental, whole mouth	10–30	1	0
chest film	5–10	1	1
abdominal films	1,150	110	25–120
spine films	1,100–2,200	85–165	22–300
kidney films (IVP)	500–1,500	75	60–130
upper GI series	400–1,300	34	12–80
barium enema	500–2,500	630	175–500
CT scan	2,000–6,000	data not given	data not given

In addition, special studies using isotopes can produce enormous specific-organ exposure: liver scan (1,500 millirems), thyroid (80,000 millirems).

Admittedly, there are instances when X-ray and isotope examinations are vital. Still, several studies have shown that 20 percent to 30 percent of radiologic tests are superfluous. For that reason, alert consumers might consider these suggestions:

Determine if a particular test is necessary. If it isn't, don't have it. Purely routine X rays are rarely indicated. Certain examinations, like gallbladder series, have been superseded by newer, less dangerous procedures.

Insist that you have your X-ray exams performed in a facility where equipment is new and the doctors are using modern high-speed film. Once installed, X-ray machines need not be checked for hazard, so films made in a doctor's office may be made on outmoded machines whose spillage can produce unwanted excess danger.

Make sure that you are shielded with lead barriers during the procedure. Scatter radiation can be lethal to tissues like thyroid, bone marrow in the breastbone, breasts and reproductive organs.

Refuse fluoroscopy, wide fields and multiple views, unless you can be convinced that the additional exposure is absolutely necessary.

Demand to know whether alternative techniques, like magnetic resonance and ultrasound, could be used instead of conventional radiation. In particular, *parents must not accept, as a matter of faith, radiological tests on their children.* Such tests, especially CT scans, are often not indicated. The risk of radiation exposure is high in children because of the cumulative effects of repeated exposure.

Although doctors owe their patients accurate diagnosis, the medical profession has the equally serious responsibility of protecting us from harmful tests. In all circumstances, adopt the aggressive position: is that X ray necessary?

Despite what many doctors believe, an informed consumer makes the best patient. Even though you may trust your physician, you should still question any medical test and weigh the risk/benefit ratio. For example, a complete blood count (CBC) is entirely safe. There is slight discomfort from the blood drawing and a small fee for the performance of the study. But to my knowledge, nobody has ever become ill or died from a routine blood test. The benefits of the test far exceed the risks.

On the other hand, X-ray examinations are in a different category. They require that the patient be placed in a beam of radiation while high-energy particles penetrate his body. Although the effects of small doses—say, the 10 millirems of a chest film—are probably insignificant, these effects are cumulative: the more X rays, the greater the likelihood of normal tissue disruption. Furthermore, some otherwise normal persons are more susceptible than others to the effects of radiation. Since there is a risk from X-ray exposure, the risk/benefit ratio must be carefully analyzed.

Years ago, no one realized the dangers of X rays. You could go into any shoe store, put your foot under a fluoroscope, press a button, and watch your toe bones wiggle. You couldn't feel or see the X rays, so they obviously couldn't hurt you. Now we know that in those early days thousands of adults and children, not to mention the poor salesmen who were constantly exposed to scatter, received unacceptable amounts of radiation. We acted out of ignorance.

Since then, scientists have progressively lowered the "acceptable" dose of radiation. Today, there is concern that even low-dose radiation may not be safe. We must not jeopardize our health because of incomplete knowledge.

It's no secret that people living on mountaintops around the world have a higher incidence of cancer than those residing at sea level. This phenomenon is thought to be due to the elevated levels of chronic, naturally occurring cosmic radiation that reaches mountain dwellers who are not as well protected by the atmosphere as are lowlanders.

Nonetheless, we are assured by many doctors—some of whom rely on X rays for their livelihoods—that medical X rays are "perfectly safe." On what criteria do these authorities base their opinions? Remember, yesterday's experts distributed primitive fluoroscopes to shoe stores.

The fact is, we don't know what is safe. Until the definitive experiments have been reported and we have unequivocal answers, the thinking consumer, it seems to me, must remain skeptical. I am not suggesting that medical and dental X-ray exams be abolished. I am urging caution. Opinions change, new hazards are defined, and what we think is safe often turns out to be dangerous.

As a rule, most X-ray tests are helpful and provide necessary information that enables people to lead more healthful, comfortable lives. Blind and unquestioned faith, however, is better suited to religion than to medicine. Patients must ask questions and expect honest answers. The risk/benefit ratio is a valuable concept, a first cousin to common sense. Let's utilize it so that in twenty years, we won't be in the position of sneering at the shoe-store physicians of the 1980s.

WE ARE WILDLY OVER-MEDICATED

❖

Judging from an enormous array of available medicines, Americans— and, I believe, most people in the civilized world—take drugs pretty much as a matter of routine. Put another way, we tend to rely on medication to get us through most illnesses, both inconsequential and serious. This approach may have important drawbacks.

Unquestionably, science has provided—and continues to provide— truly remarkable antidotes to disease. We are all aware of a biochemical revolution that started in the 1930s with the discovery of antibiotics. The initial, tentative, lapping ripples of success have progressed to tidal waves of discovery; vaccination, improved forms of old medicine, beta blockers, anticancer drugs, calcium channel blockers. We are now at the threshold of an extraordinary new era. Biochemists are beginning to concoct new potions that affect only very specific portions of our chemical makeup to prevent, control or cure disease. In the future, drug therapy will almost certainly consist of highly purified medicines, virtually free of side effects. However, we need constant reminding that such a therapeutic nirvana isn't here yet. Currently available medications produce many complications. In our joyful rush to cure our ills by swallowing pills, we must exercise caution and retain a healthy skepticism.

To begin with, every bona fide drug has side effects. Sometimes these effects are minor; often they are not. For example, although aspirin causes intestinal bleeding in *each* person who takes it, the beneficial consequences of the medicine usually outweigh this complication. For some people, however, aspirin can cause serious and life-threatening reactions like asthma and uncontrolled bleeding.

Any chemical that is useful as a medicine causes unwanted repercussions. The more powerful the drug, the greater the chance of serious side effects. I am not referring to unusual allergic manifestations. I am talking about a drug's normal unwanted results: everything from impotence to anemia. These reactions occur with regularity.

I have identified two interesting phenomena in my own practice: 1. About 75 percent of the medicines I now regularly prescribe had not been developed when I was in medical school. 2. A hefty percentage of patients, particularly the elderly, are being poisoned by the drugs they take. People are wildly overmedicated. Most doctors routinely prescribe one compound to counteract the effects of another; the most common, I suspect, is the use of supplemental potassium to replace losses from diuretics.

Many medicines simply do not blend well in people, and I defy any physician who insists on multiple-drug regimens to keep track of what is reacting with what. The recent reports of broccoli interfering with the effectiveness of blood anticoagulants should be enough to make any practitioner shudder. Put simply, we doctors are not smart enough to predict all the drug interactions that can take place. Even diet (no milk products with tetracycline), alcohol (affects almost any medication) and smoking (increases tendency of the blood to clot) can cause far-reaching effects in the pill taker.

In the second place, what about the risk of death from medicine? Well, we all play the numbers on this one. If a single person in 100,000 will die from taking a certain drug, we shrug and say it can't be me... or my patient. In fact, what are the statistical chances of death? *We* don't know, and since we have no method of predicting such a bizarre and unusual event, every patient is at risk. If he takes a pill, he may live—or be the one in 100,000 who dies. No wonder the thoughtful physician worries about each patient under treatment.

Medicines are necessary. They usually do what they are supposed to do. But we had better know what we want to accomplish when we take drugs. Here is an area where doctor and patient can really work together: the former by an honest appraisal of what is necessary, the latter by understanding the potential consequences through thorough questioning.

MEGA-WOES OF MEGA-VITAMINS

❖

For adults, when it comes to giving medicine, the old saying used to be: "Two pills for a horse, one for a man." Among some consumers, this aphorism has been expanded so that, when taking vitamins, "the more the better."

Vitamins are currently in vogue. In some quarters, they are looked upon as cure-alls, panaceas to correct everything from depression and boredom to falling hair and cracked lips. Some vitamin proponents believe that massive doses, "megaitamin therapy," can cure mental illness, treat drug addiction and modify antisocial behavior.

In fact, while vitamins are important ingredients of a well-balanced diet, they are not new wonder drugs able to leap the tall buildings of human disease. Nor are they faster than speeding bullets or more powerful than locomotives. Quite simply, they are trace compounds necessary for the normal function of living tissue. "Megadoses" of vitamins have not been proven scientifically to be more beneficial to us than are plain old small doses, carefully calculated by continued experimentation, and administered as the Recommended Daily Allowance (RDA) to prevent or correct deficiencies. If the infatuation with megavitamin therapy has had any fallout, it is the modern demonstration that—like any nutritional constituent—vitamins can produce toxic effects if taken indiscriminately in large doses for long periods of time.

Vitamin A, in therapeutic quantities (800 to 1,000 retinol equivalents), is necessary to prevent night blindness and to maintain normal growth of tissues. Doses that exceed the RDA can produce headaches, nausea, vomiting, skin shedding, hair loss, fatigue, hemorrhage, disorientation, liver enlargement and bone pain.

Niacin is essential for energy metabolism. The RDA is 13 to 19 niacin equivalents. Overdose can cause skin flushing, heart-rhythm disturbances, headache, cramps, vomiting, diarrhea, elevated blood sugar, peptic ulcer and gout.

Vitamin B is required for amino-acid metabolism and formation of red blood cells. The RDA is about 2 mg. Excessive ingestion of pyridoxine produces nerve damage in legs and arms, seizures and peptic disease. B_6 decreases the effect of the medicine L-dopa, so the vitamin is contraindicated in patients being treated with this drug for Parkinson's disease.

Vitamin B_{12} prevents pernicious anemia and is probably the safest vitamin. The RDA is 2 micrograms, but no adverse effects are seen with much higher doses. But in cancer patients taking methotrexate, adverse interaction with B_{12} can occur.

Vitamin C, with an RDA of 60 mg., plays a role in maintaining body tissues, including white blood cells. No responsible investigations have shown that high doses protect against the common cold or any infection. In fact, massive doses may cause B_{12} deficiency, iron overload, diarrhea, kidney stones and breakdown of red blood cells. Ascorbic acid interferes with a variety of laboratory tests and can interact with anticoagulant drugs. Rebound scurvy has been reported in women who suddenly stopped taking megadoses.

Vitamin D is necessary for healthy bones. The RDA is 200 to 400 international units. Chronic overdose can produce nausea, vomiting, diarrhea, headache, weight loss, weakness, fatigue, confusion, kidney failure, calcium deposits in kidneys, bone pain, cramps, excessive blood calcium and increased risk of heart attacks.

Vitamin E is an antioxidant. Its precise role in the body is not completely understood. The RDA is 8 to 10 international units. The vitamin is useful in treating visual loss in certain premature infants and may be helpful in reducing painful breast lumpiness in women. Excessive doses have been reported to cause weakness, blood clots, high blood pressure, elevated blood sugar, nausea and fatigue. The vitamin enhances the effects of anticoagulants.

Vitamin K is vital for normal blood coagulation. The RDA is 70 to 140 micrograms. Toxicity is rare but can be seen as hemorrhage, kidney degeneration, liver damage and anemia.

Thiamine enhances the metabolism of certain amino acids. The RDA is 1 to 1.5 mg. Large doses, given intramuscularly by injection, can cause nausea, difficulty in breathing and rapid heart rate.

The preceding synopsis is based on valid medical investigations. If a consumer chooses to accept, in preference, noncientific claims based on unproved opinion and anecdote, he risks potential self-inflicted hazard.

With vitamins—and indeed, all medicine—more is not necessarily better.

MEET THE KILLER TISSUE

I was amused to discover some time ago a new nadir of American ingenuity: Avert, by Kleenex, a tissue marketed to kill cold-causing viruses while you blow.

With the enthusiasm ordinarily reserved for drug companies introducing death-defying potions, Kimberly-Clark heralds Avert as "virucidal." When you blow your nose into the thing, chemicals in the impregnated paper will magically wipe out nasty germs, including those that cause influenza. You now have the power to avoid contaminating your family with the actively infectious virus residue that dribbles onto your hands each time you blow, cough or sneeze.

The manufacturer of this artifice encourages you to "use liberally" for colds and flu. No doubt that's good advice: you'd have to use a truckload to do any good.

I really want to understand this. I am making an effort, so please bear with me. Avert makes use of citric acid from grapefruit, lauryl sulfate (an ingredient of toothpaste) and something called malic acid, from God knows where, all of which act in a second or two to maim viruses that threaten your loved ones. You may feel miserable, since nothing can cure your cold, but you can rest easy in the knowledge that "viruses that are stopped on the tissue can't be spread to others."

If this were true, I wouldn't be surprised to learn that flu sufferers were stuffing the things up their noses or chewing them like Bull Durham. With all the pain and devastation in the world—famine, child abuse, uncontrollable diseases, acid rain and threat of nuclear demolition—has American industry finally succeeded, where others have failed, in achieving a public-health breakthrough?

Or is this, as I suspect, just another promotional gimmick to sell more Kleenex?

I must confess that I actually know—yes, can identify, under threat of torture—people who still use handkerchiefs. I also know people who don't, but they're a topic more suitable for another essay. Through recorded history, perfectly law-abiding handkerchief users have been selfishly oblivious of the epidemics they are spreading. Isn't it marvelous that at last we have been rescued from abysmal ignorance? Like public toilet seats, our respiratory secretions can now be realistically viewed in the proper perspective: malevolent dangers reflecting the many risks of overcrowding in a technological society.

The cynic might be tempted to suggest that a federal program to instruct all citizens in how to blow their noses might be a more cost-effective method of combating the terrors of rhinoviruses type 1A. I've noted that children, in particular, tend to blow only when told. Will the miracle of Avert revolutionize the classic caricature of snotty-nosed schoolchildren? Unlikely. Perhaps grapefruit toothpaste would be a more efficient virus eradicator.

We educated adults are being brainwashed into believing that all body secretions are malignant drools that can destroy us. Nature needs improving. What we can't sanitize with Lysol and Listerine, we cover with lemon freshness or peppermint. We are becoming insecure about normal body functions.

Avert exploits our national mania for cleanliness. The mania is illusory; our politics, for example, remain as dirty as ever. If you think turbocharged Kleenex with 17 percent active ingredients is going to aid you or simplify your life, you'll believe anything. Thank heaven the product, like the medical profession, contains 83 percent *inactive* ingredients.

We all would like to remain healthy. But using virucidal facial tissues is, at best, a doubtful method of achieving this goal. The product probably will enjoy moderate success because it emphasizes our preoccupation with being more acceptable and attractive. You can't possibly be rejected if you smell good, shine, say the right things and use impregnated Kleenex—no matter that you can't dance or read, are a klutz, and venerate *The Dukes of Hazzard* as an allegory of the human condition.

It's been said that, in this country, you first make the product and then develop the market. We've been inundated by past specimens: electric carving knives, computer dating, the pet rock, air fresheners and breakfast cereal shot from guns. We adore novelty. But in our blind acceptance of superficially appealing products, we must remember not to be intimidated by slick salesmanship. Virucidal tissues are one of the latest, but by no means the last, efforts by industry to make a profit by pandering to our distrust of ourselves.

If you don't agree with my position, that's okay. Now let's talk about scented toilet paper...

HIDDEN ALCOHOL IN OUR MEDICINES

Years ago, health tonics were widely believed to be beneficial agents that helped cure disease. They made people feel better. They were popular over-the-counter medications.

Tonics have been replaced now with new formulas. When it was discovered that alcohol was the major ingredient in many tonics, the public turned away from those old-fashioned brews. Yet elixirs and tonics are still very much with us—under different names.

Today's products are marketed primarily for coughs, colds and congestion. They contain new chemicals, but the chemicals are still diluted with alcohol. More than five hundred proprietary medications contain alcohol in concentrations of up to 68 percent (136 proof). Many are liquid vitamin mixtures.

This alcohol is not innocuous. It can increase gastric acidity, depress brain function and produce dangerous reactions in recovering alcoholics. Of more potential importance are the long-term effects of administering alcohol-containing compounds to young children.

Prescription drugs may contain alcohol—for example: Donnatal Elixir (23 percent alcohol, plus phenobarbital), Elixophyllin Elixir (20 percent alcohol), Quibron Elixir (15 percent), Benadryl Elixir (14 percent), Propadrine Elixir (16 percent) and Terpin Hydrate Elixir (24 percent).

More significantly, common nonprescription liquid preparations contain high concentrations of alcohol: Dristan (12 percent), Nyquil (25 percent), Vicks 44 (10 percent) and Geritol (12 percent). Children are frequently given Novahistine Expectorant (5 percent), Phenergan Expectorant (7 percent), Tylenol Elixir (7 percent) and Cheracol (3 percent).

Here are some other preparations, listed with alcohol content:

Alurate Elixir (20 percent), Amytal Elixir (30 percent), Bentyl-PB syrup (19 percent), Broncho-Tussin (40 percent), Cenalene Elixir (15 percent), Choledyl Elixir (20 percent), Coldene Elixir (adult; 15 percent), Creo-Terpin (25 percent), Dexamyl Elixir (25 percent), Dolanex Elixir (23 percent), Elixodyne (20 percent), Geriplex-FS (18 percent), Gerix Elixir (20 percent), Gevrabon (18 percent), Hybephen Elixir (16.5 percent), Isuprel Compound Elixir (19 percent), Keralyt (19.4 percent), Lanoxin Pediatric Elixir (10 percent), Lomotil Liquid (15 percent), Lufyllin Elixir (20 percent), Mini-lix Elixir (20 percent), Mundrane G.G. Elixir (20 percent), Norophylline (20 percent), Organidin Elixir (24 percent), Peri-Colace Syrup (10 percent), Pertussin Plus (25 percent), Prolixin Elixir (14 percent), Synophylate Elixir (20 percent), Theo-Guaia (20 percent), Theon Elixir (28 percent), Uritone Elixir (20 percent), Valarian (68 percent).

Many consumers are concerned about the overuse of alcohol in medicines. Fortunately, many reputable drug companies share this concern and are manufacturing alcohol-free medicines. Some common liquid medicines that contain no alcohol are : Actifed-C Expectorant, Codimal Expectorant, Conar-A, Glycotuss Syrup, Hycomine Pediatric Syrup, Omni-Tuss Suspension, Pyribenzamine Expectorant, Romex, Silence Is Golden Cough Syrup, Sorbase Cough Syrup, Triaminicol Cough Syrup and Tussionex Suspension.

You may ask: What purpose is served by this boring index of medication? The answer is: I believe we need to know what constituents of medicine we feed ourselves and our children. One tablespoon of a 20-percent alcohol preparation is the equivalent of one ounce of wine. If a patient wants an alcohol-free medicine, he or she should have access to the necessary information. The recent reports that some so-called "alcohol-free" beers actually contain alcohol (albeit in amounts of less than 0.5 percent) focuses attention on labels that are misleading or downright dishonest.

A two- or three-teaspoon dose of a cough medicine containing alcohol can be quite a belt for youngsters. Even the sound sleep, so popularized in TV ads, that results from the use of an over-the-counter adult cold remedy may be due more to the alcohol content than the supposedly active ingredients. This type of medicine can be disastrous for a person who is trying to kick a drinking habit.

Therefore, know what you want, read labels on medicine bottles and check with your doctor. Even better, check with your pharmacist. This is the kind of information he or she is trained to provide.

EATING WHAT COMES "NATURALLY"

❖

"Natural" foods are enjoying (as much as any food can enjoy anything) a boom in popularity. Diet faddists, health-food advocates and plain old consumers are increasingly grasping at foods with "natural ingredients." Part of the swing away from processed foods undoubtedly comes from the genuine fear we all have that, somehow, manufactured edibles contain chemicals and contaminants damaging to the human body. I would guess that even the most indifferent person believes, all things considered, that fresh food that has not been monkeyed with is "better." Agreed? Think of all the hormones in meat, artificial sweeteners and colorings, the sodium this-and-that added for freshness, the nitrate to retard spoilage, refined sugar that makes holes in teeth and hearts. We must be demented to shove that stuff into our maltreated, unsuspecting gastrointestinal tracts. Let's get back to natural foods, and know what we are eating. Never mind that the fresh lettuce may have been sprayed with insecticides, the milk laced with radioactive material from Russian nuclear disasters, the fresh fish a reservoir for mercury and horrendous chemicals.

It didn't take the food industry long to accommodate our

wishes. Labels dutifully indicate ingredients. One case in point: yogurt. How can a manufacturer foul up something as simple as yogurt? That's what a pharmacist in Boston wondered as he casually read the list of ingredients on a container of "natural" cherry yogurt he was happily finishing. His eyes stopped at the innocuous name "cochineal," a natural food coloring. A bell rang in his intracranial steeple and he researched the "natural" ingredient. Here is what he found. Cochineal consists of dried insects. The female of the species lays her eggs, then promptly dies and covers them with her dead body. These bugs are cultivated on cactuses in tropical America where they are gathered—dead bloated females with waxy hides, covering eggs and hatched larvae—and shipped to the United States for use as food coloring. You see, the egg yolks and fatty parts of the adult females are—you guessed it—red.

Although the Food and Drug Administration recognizes the filthy nature of the red glop and specifies treatment to destroy typhoidlike bacteria, it makes no provisions to eliminate other bacteria or toxins possibly present in the mush. The cochineal is eventually added to "All Natural Black Cherry Flavored Yogurt," and heaven knows what other foods.

So, there you are. It's either BHA-BHT, Red Dye #2 or a squashed red bug resembling a wood louse. Natural ingredients, currently the fad, may have their own problems. Cool Whip, anyone?

MODERN SNAKE-OIL SALESMEN

❖

Medical quackery has been reported to be a $25-billion national scandal. The traveling snake-oil salesman, hawking his wares from the back of a horse-drawn wagon, has been supplanted by the no-less-greedy entrepreneur who uses modern marketing techniques to separate the sucker from his dollar.

Only about 1 percent of the Food and Drug Administration's budget goes to fight quackery. According to a Washington *Post* story in 1985, federal authorities are hamstrung by the enormity of the lucrative business. Dr. Victor Herbert, professor of medicine at the Hahnemann Medical Center in Philadelphia, is an expert on nutrition and health fraud. He has called for a Task Force on Health Quackery to step up prosecution against a problem that has reached the proportions of organized crime.

Promoters are not only clever, but will go to almost any extreme to bilk a naïve public. An astounding amount of money is spent by ordinary citizens on pure trash. "Moon dust," an alleged arthritis cure that cost $30 an ounce, turned out to be common sand. The "miracle spike" cost $300, was supposed to cure cancer and diabetes, and was found to contain several cents' worth of rat poison. The microdynameter, at $900, was touted as a cure for virtually any disease; it consisted of a galvanometer attached to electrodes that would stimulate the skin.

Unregulated health foods are flooding the market in a billion-dollar rip-off. Mexican clinics, offering untested and dangerous "secret" drugs, milk millions of U.S. dollars from sick people desperate for remedies. The cosmetic industry is burgeoning, in part because of skin creams that promise the user a youthful appearance. Dr. Sorrel Schwartz, professor of pharmacology at

Georgetown University, wryly observes that "anybody 60 years old who believes something he takes is going to give him the skin of a 20-year-old probably deserves what he gets." The professor says that medical quackery extends "from the ridiculous and the almost-funny to the tragic. It runs the gamut from people who don't have enough intelligence to void in the morning to people with M.D. degrees." Representative Claude Pepper (D-Fla.) commented: "We found the inventiveness of quacks to be as unlimited as their callousness and greed. There are so many opportunities for quackery. The human heart yearns for health and happiness, and therefore is gullible."

If quackery stems from people's most urgent and fundamental desire to feel better, then it seems to me that quacks can be put out of business only by the very public they exploit. Laws and legislation may help, but in the final analysis, it's our problem. Civilization has probably been plagued by charlatans since before recorded history. You would assume that as we have become more discerning and sophisticated, we would exercise more discrimination. Alas, this appears not to be so. The quacks have become more sophisticated, too.

Despite its many drawbacks and flaws, traditional medicine has one thing going for it: In any culture, it usually represents a distillation of the wisdom of the finest thinkers of the tribe. What gives modern traditional medicine such an edge is the scientific method; without objective analysis and proof, any tradition is no more than a myth. If modern medical techniques have revolutionized the approach to and management of disease, it is because of hard work, scrupulousness and constant reassessment—not because of vapid claims and hollow promises.

If we are to survive in our complex society, we must remain skeptical in a constructive and intelligent way. We must question, demand proof and rely on our experience of the real world. If we allow ourselves to be exploited by promoters of outrageous schemes, we will not have progressed beyond our earliest ancestors, who howled at the moon, made sacrifices to the sun god and hid in terror because they regarded an eclipse as the end of the world.

**FAST
FOODS**

❖

Fifty thousand fast-food restaurants in this country constitute a multibillion-dollar industry. The popularity of such food is staggering, and is unlikely to diminish. Fast foods are said to be successful because they are relatively inexpensive, quickly prepared, predictably unvaried and hunger-satisfying. Because fast foods appear increasingly to represent a large part of many Americans' diets, nutritionists have expressed alarm over the nutritional deficiencies of fast foods and the potential health problems fast-food consumers risk developing.

A typical fast-food meal contains 900 to 1,300 calories, about half the daily caloric requirement of an adult male. The calories are derived chiefly from the high fat and carbohydrate contents of these foods. Grilled and fried foods have unusually high caloric levels, as do thick shakes, which are made with powdered milk, vegetable fats and sweetening agents. For the overweight person, these meals may be a disaster. So too must fast foods be avoided by the cholesterol-conscious consumer. The recent disclosure that some of our most popular fast-food chains fry their food in beef fat is additional cause for alarm. The high-fat diet enjoyed by many Americans may predispose them—even children—to premature hardening of the arteries. Fast foods may contribute to this trend.

Fast-food meals usually contain adequate protein (25–72 grams). However, these foods are lacking in crude fiber, iron and vitamins—notably, A, D, C, B_{12} and thiamine. Because of its cheese content, pizza is high in calcium; other fast foods (except milk shakes) do not supply much of this mineral.

Inexpensive as they may seem, fast-food meals are easy to prepare at home and would cost less if they were. For example,

McDonald's hamburgers cost about one-third more than the home-prepared equivalent; McDonald's apple pie is more than three times as expensive as its homemade counterpart. In general, restaurant food costs about twice as much as food prepared at home.

The menus in fast-food chains tend to be predictably monotonous. Therefore, regular outings can adversely influence developing food preferences in children who may not learn to enjoy a healthy variety but may substitute cholesterol-laden, calorie-rich food for nutritious fare. Fortunately, some food chains are now heavily advertising appealing breakfasts. For people who ordinarily omit breakfast, this campaign should have beneficial effects.

The consumer is lured to fast-food restaurants by advertising. Hundreds of millions of dollars have been spent in a successful effort to persuade us all that fast food is as American as apple pie. The stuff is available in supermarkets, vending machines, schools, zoos—even hospitals!

Despite the fact that, more than ever, Americans want to learn about nutrition and healthy living, fast foods have come to be so ubiquitous that many diners are regularly compromising health to worship at the altar of sweet taste and speedy service. Like detective stories and grade-B movies, fast food has a role in our society. But reason dictates that we give equal time to serious novels, art films and fresh vegetables.

The average family has been estimated to eat out four to seven times a week. That figure seems high to me. Few people I know eat at restaurants that often. Like drinking in a bar, eating out is much more expensive and, in the case of fast-food restaurants, less nutritious than eating at home. But *somebody* is spending the more than $6 billion a year on Whoppers, Buster Bars, Big Macs, Peg Legs and Bell Beefers. Just one taste of that glop should be enough to send anyone running to the fresh-food department of the local grocery store. It's enough to gag a maggot.

Fortunately, strong consumer pressure is being exerted on manufacturers of prepared foods to list the nutrient composition of their wares. Fast food must be supplemented by a varied and balanced intake of more nourishing, less saturated, less fattening edibles that have not been processed to death.

CUTTING CORNERS IN MEDICINE

❖

Remember the film *The China Syndrome*? It was an eloquent testimonial to one man's stand against a society in which "cutting corners" had become a national preoccupation. The movie depicted an assistant supervisor of a nuclear power plant who loses his life in part because he is willing to reveal publicly that quality control of welded seams in a cooling pump had been dangerously compromised. When confronted with the evidence of wrongdoing, the inspector defends his deception by stating that "everybody" has to cut corners.

We don't need Jane Fonda and Hollywood to remind us that we live in a cutting-corners culture. Take a close look at your new appliance or automobile. I'll be surprised if you don't find faults directly attributable to workmen who compromised quality. It's no myth that cars assembled on Mondays and Fridays are inferior to those made during midweek shifts. Doing things more easily or automatically has wrongly become synonymous with cutting corners.

Unfortunately, medicine is not immune to this collective mentality. The public is, of course, well aware of this. Although doctors delude themselves by pretending it isn't so, many patients recognize and object to this disturbing trend.

In essence, some physicians and surgeons have adopted the policy of administering less care while charging routine and customary fees. An occasional doctor will grossly overcharge. The rationale? "Well, Medicare or your insurance will pay the bill, so don't worry."

A lot of people are worrying, however, because not only is this corner cutting morally reprehensible, it unquestionably increases our tax burden and insurance premiums. In all fairness, I emphasize that this practice is restricted to only a small portion of doctors. Nonetheless, as with nuclear power plants, a handful of corner cutters can jeopardize the reputation of the whole profession. What can you, the consumer, do to avoid becoming a victim of medical corner cutting?

To begin with, ask questions of your doctor before he provides a service. What are his usual charges for an office call? A particular procedure? An operation? Do his surgical fees cover work he performs immediately before surgery? Follow-up visits? What "extras" can you reasonably expect to be charged for? What is the approximate cost of whatever tests you may require? Does he charge more for special attention and intensive care? How much? Why? Can you both work out an appropriate flat-fee arrangement before he provides services?

Naturally, these questions would not necessarily be asked prior to emergency services, when the only priority is the saving of life. However, if you have a family physician or personal doctor, you can query him about his charges for emergency services before they are required. Does he make house calls if needed? How much would he charge for a middle-of-the-night house call or an emergency-room evaluation? What are his hourly charges both during and after office hours? If you don't agree with what your doctor tells you about his fees, you have every right to talk to other doctors, to get a clearer idea of the prevailing fees in your community.

Let's suppose you have been unwilling or unable to ask questions and now find yourself the recipient of a large medical bill (which may or may not be taken care of by insurance). What are your options?

First, you can write to your doctor and ask for a reduction. If he refuses to comply or allows an inconsequential reduction, you may then write the details of your complaint to the executive committee or the grievance committee of the county medical society to which your doctor belongs. If he doesn't belong to a county or state medical association, beware. The committee will review your complaint and possibly talk to your doctor in an attempt to encourage him to reduce his bill. The committee may then ask you and the doctor to appear in person to explain your disagreement.

If satisfactory resolutions still cannot be reached, the committee will canvass other doctors in the county to determine if the fee was customary or whether it was excessive. If the fee was excessive, the committee can usually exert pressure on the doctor to make a "voluntary" reduction. Failing this, there are various legal alternatives available to you and the committee. Although these alternatives vary among states and their medical societies, it is infrequent that an eventual agreement cannot be concluded.

In any case, you—the patient—are not at the mercy of the System. You have the right to fair consideration; recourse is available. Alert and cost-conscious consumers are the best answer to the epidemic of corner cutting in industry and the infrequent but disturbing cases in the medical profession. We must all take more active roles in controlling the quality of life in our environment. If we do, we can avoid the equivalent of a Three Mile Island disaster in medicine.

AN EXPERT DIAGNOSIS

❖

I've stopped telling my auto mechanic what is wrong with my car. One day last spring, I learned a thing or two about diagnosis.

The engine of my little vintage sports car was running very unevenly; actually, it wasn't running, it was limping. By the time I arrived at the repair shop, it was crawling on its knees, huffing and wheezing like a patient with emphysema. Against a background of *poop-wheeze-poop-bop* from the car, I held a discussion with the mechanic.

"Trouble, Doc?" (Smiles. Wipes his hands. Peers intently under the upraised bonnet.)

"Yeah, Doug. I think the timing's shot."

"Hmmm. Doesn't sound like that's the problem."

"Could it be a fouled spark plug?"

"Maybe." (He begins to remove what I think is the air filter.)

"Water in the gas?"

"Could be." (Pause.) "Look, Doc, please do me a favor. Just tell me the symptoms. Let me make the diagnosis."

"Okay. The car's been garaged for the winter. When I started it up, the engine caught, it idled and then began to miss."

"Well!" (Triumphant.) "Here's the problem." (He holds the air filter in his hands. Nestled in the baffles is a large mouse nest filled with string, fuzz, seedpods, droppings and a variety of materials used by the tiny ubiquitous rodents that continue to invade my life at inopportune times.)

"It's the mice!"

"Sure is. They were in the filter for months. Engine couldn't get enough air." (He removes massive amounts of lint from the carburetor intake, and the engine begins to burble and purr.)

"Thanks, Doug."

"Don't mention it. Remember, Doc, let me do the diagnosing."

I was chastened by that experience and subsequently became quite adept at describing car problems to mechanics. Sometimes my descriptions are sufficient to enable the repairmen to tell me, on the telephone, how to correct the malfunction (for example, by cleaning the battery terminals).

During my years in medical practice, I've come to realize that fixing cars can sometimes be akin to fixing people. Professionals in both fields are trained to interpret signs and symptoms. Using an organized and (usually) rational process, mechanics and doctors sift and evaluate, examine and test, in order to define treatment. In both occupations, there are simple problems that are obvious, regular checkups, diagnostic dilemmas, specialists, cosmetic procedures, increasing reliance on electronic gadgets, serious conditions requiring major overhauls, problems of abuse and aging. Unfortunately, there are unscrupulous mechanics who, like some doctors, are interested primarily in maximizing profits. But most, like most doctors, are honest and dependable.

In my office, when patients open discussions by telling me their diagnosis, I often gently remind them, as Doug reminded me, to tell me their symptoms and let me do the diagnosing. They should feel comfortable about asking me any questions that are on their minds and describing fully what is troubling them, but Doug was right—presenting him with a diagnosis before he had a chance to investigate on his own just wasn't helpful.

I have a lot of respect for automobile mechanics. They are brothers in the cloth. They probably have as much trouble as I do collecting from insurance companies. They certainly have as much paper work and the headache of dealing with government agencies. They are expected to be available at all hours. They can make our lives much more comfortable and enjoyable. I think they would make good doctors. And they sure as heck would be less expensive.

HARRY'S CONSUMER COMA

Lawyers who orchestrate patients' million-dollar malpractice suits stress that doctors must place greater emphasis on explaining to people the limits, extent, and complications of medical testing and treatment. Plaintiffs' attorneys point out that the basis for negligence claims is simply that the doctor did not provide to the patient sufficient information about the potential consequences of a medical or surgical act. That is, the physician did not give "informed consent."

I do not know a single M.D. who does not agree with this principle. We try to explain things. However, like many issues in life, the question is one of degree. I'll give you an example.

Here is a sixty-three-year-old man with a two-day illness characterized by fever of 102 degrees, achiness, scratchy throat, headache, sore joints, upset stomach, and occasional hacking cough. He is usually in good health and has no history of ulcer, lung problems or heart disease.

I have talked to at least two dozen adults with similar symptoms in the past week. It is the flu season, and I suspect my patient has a self-limited virus infection that will run its course in about three days. Nonetheless, because of his age, I make a house call. He has a fever. His nose is runny, and his throat is blotchy red. There are no signs of arthritis, heart failure, pneumonia or meningitis. I say: "Look, Harry, I think you've got the flu. I doubt that you have a serious condition. Stay quiet, drink lots of fluids, take a couple of aspirin every four hours if your fever goes above ninety-nine degrees, and call me on Thursday."

This sounds like a reasonable approach to me, and Harry seems content with my analysis. I think I have done my job: established a diagnosis by exclusion, suggested a conservative approach and arranged for follow-up. The transaction appears satisfactorily complete. I have fulfilled my role as a physician and addressed the problem with minimal expense.

I'm taking a big risk in doing this, though, because I've based my actions on clinical judgment instead of extensive testing. If I were practicing "defensive medicine," an increasingly prevalent abhorrence, I would do more. Not for Harry's sake, you understand, but for my own. I'd have to cover any liability that could arise and anticipate unusual contingencies so I wouldn't end up in court. I would order a blood count to make sure that Harry had enough infection-fighting blood cells. After all, he could have leukemia. I'd obtain two chest X rays (front and side) to rule out a small area of pneumonia. I might insist on a urinalysis to cover the unlikely possibility of kidney infection. I'd get a throat culture to see if he has a strep. I might even go further with a cardiogram and a complete blood chemical-screening battery. All of a sudden, a $24 case of grippe balloons into a $200 extravaganza. Is the purpose of this fishing expedition to discover the unusual disease? Partially; primarily, it is to protect me from getting sued.

Even if the tests are normal, I'm not off the hook. You see, I didn't give Harry a thorough rundown about the possible consequences of taking aspirin. Had I done so, here is how my comments would be revised: "Harry, I think aspirin will bring down your fever and make you feel better. However, there are potential dangers of aspirin that are listed by the manufacturer. The drug can cause fatal allergic reactions that may cause you to go into shock. It may affect the coagulation of your blood so that you could bleed to death. It may give you heartburn, gas, vomiting, ulcers, stomach bleeding, and massive gastrointestinal hemorrhage. It can trigger asthma. You may experience ringing in your ears. Keep this and all medicines out of the reach of children. In case of accidental overdose, consult your physician immediately. The medicine is to be used only for temporary relief of discomfort and fever resulting from colds and flu, sore throats, muscular aches and pains, arthritis, bursitus, rheumatism, lumbago, sciatica, toothache, neuralgia, menstrual pain, sleeplessness and pain accompanying immunizations. You may experience nervousness, dizziness and sleepiness. Do not use in the presence of high blood pressure, heart disease, diabetes, or thyroid disorders. Do you have any questions? Good. Please sign this consent form in which you acknowledge that you fully accept the risks of aspirin therapy and that these consequences have been fully explained to you in understandable terms. Mrs. Miller will witness and notarize this document."

By now, Harry is in the advanced stages of consumer coma, which has nothing to do with the flu. He would probably be content to curl up in bed, clutching his medical bills, and suffer—rather than risk death or incapacitation from aspirin. Can you imagine the extent to which I'd have to go if the patient had a serious condition requiring surgery or more potent medication? As I said earlier, it's a matter of degree.

CHAPTER 8

EASE
AND
DIS-EASE

HOW
NOT TO

❖

HOW–TO is in and has been with us now for quite a while. If you want to publish a book, simply write a manual on how to do something. After jet-set romances and executive autobiographies, how-to books are still among the hottest items on bookstore shelves.

I'm not referring to books describing the development of skills, such as How to Build Your Own House or How to Macrame with Fishing Tackle. I allude to how-to books about *personal* stuff like . . . well . . . your *life*.

These books cover a wide range of topics: how to eat; how not to eat; how to drink alcohol and eat less; how to walk, run, exercise; how not to exercise; how to make love, make a million, make more of yourself, make less of yourself and more of others; how to make believe; how to get rid of your husband, pimples, Dutch elm disease; how to cope with the anxiety of impending nuclear war; and how to cope with having a baby, a bitchy mother, shin splints, bad dreams, hemorrhoids . . . I could go on and on.

To look at the lists of books telling us what to do and how to do it, you would think we had become a nation of incompetent nincompoops. When I was growing up, the only how-to book I remember was written by Emily Post. I never felt the need to read it, but a lot of people swore by it. Later, Dr. Spock wrote a how-to book that helped young parents who were too independent or too embarrassed to ask their own parents what to do. I don't understand how modern people can possibly assimilate the enormous amount of how-to information that is literally bursting, like overconfident spring flowers, from the bookstalls. I'm not clear how readers are expected to resolve inconsistencies and disagreements. If one book makes a statement and another book disagrees, which are we to believe? This sort of decision making puts loads of pressure on the public—pressure, I suspect, we don't need right now.

There was a time when we didn't need someone in print to tell us what to do. We ate a little of everything; we tried not to overdo. Walking and running were natural activities in which the average person did not need instruction after the age of three. If we became tired, we had the sense to stop. Have we become the victims of the books we thought we needed?

Our confidence has been sapped in an epidemic of self-doubt. We seem unable to master our everyday lives, much less our fate. What happened to old-fashioned common sense? Why do we distrust our bodies and brains? Why have we stopped listening to those small voices of propriety and good judgment that speak to us from within? Perfectly well-meaning and intelligent people often pay large sums of hard-earned money to listen to a doctor tell them what they knew all the time. It's discouraging that we have so little faith in ourselves.

Dr. Elisabeth Kubler-Ross, an acknowledged expert on death and dying, has published an illustrated book describing how certain terminally ill patients cope with their imminent deaths. It's basically a how-to book. Heaven knows, it may be a godsend: How to Die. You must admit that's not exactly a subject you can ask around about. Firsthand information is hard to obtain. So perhaps the good doctor is performing a valuable service. However, like the little field mice that refuse to leave my garage, doubts persist; they gnaw at the back of my mind. Is it possible there may be human acts so deeply personal and inalienably private that writing about them is futile and demeaning? Some of these actions do not come easily; many involve pain of one type or another. For example, a first love affair, like death, does not lend itself to book learning—even from a picture book.

I'd guess that most how-to books are purchased by people who do not trust themselves. I, for one, would like to see a return to principles of self-confidence and self-assurance. Many budding authors might then have to write real books.

LAUGHTER
AND
DISEASE

❖

There is a lot of interest these days in the relationship between disease and the psyche. Certain personality types are said to be more susceptible to specific diseases: Type A people, who choose life's fast lane, are more vulnerable to heart attacks; worry causes peptic ulcers; grief makes one prone to cancer. The popular media like to remind us that we can think our way out of disease. By changing our personalities, we can—in effect—cure ourselves.

This concept gained wide publicity after Norman Cousins reported his own self-cure of ankylosing spondylitis (a swelling of the spine and surrounding structures) using huge doses of Vitamin C—and laughter. Cousins and other articulate spokespeople are persuaded that relaxation and imagery are more than an end in themselves to foster a sense of well-being; the techniques are viewed as methods of defeating disease.

This attractive hypothesis is not new. For centuries, positive thinking has been thought to enhance mastery over our lives and to cure various afflictions. As an example, in the 1800s, tuberculosis was considered to be a disease of feeling. Passion literally "consumed" the victim. This preoccupation with emotion led to the development of the "tuberculosis-prone personality." Once the tuberculosis bacterium was isolated and identified, the disease was recognized to be an infection. The emotional theory evaporated and antibiotics were used to fight the disease.

Today, cancer, stroke and heart attack are the modern scourges. These diseases exist in epidemic proportions because no one knows what causes them. Scientists are in the process of learning more about these conditions, but cures have thus far eluded even the most ardent investigator. Past experience has taught us that magical mastery becomes a compelling component in the treatment of diseases that are incompletely understood. As a result, certain self-anointed experts prescribe for cancer patients relaxation techniques, including picturing strong white blood cells destroying weak and disorganized cancer cells.

No adult would deny that a sick person's will to survive is a beneficial adjunct to specific therapy. However, this is not to say that the total responsibility for getting well rests solely with the patient. For a variety of reasons, doctors may insidiously enhance this concept by their subtle tendency to hold the sick patient responsible for his or her own well-being. Personal failure may be a factor in some diseases, such as cigarette-induced lung cancer and drug addiction, but by the time a person has developed a serious illness, no amount of positive thinking is likely to make a significant difference in the rate or degree of cure.

In the past few months, two carefully conducted studies have cast doubt on the belief that a patient's mental state causes or cures disease. Both reports were published in the *New England Journal of Medicine*. The first showed no correlation between Type A personality and the recurrence of heart attack. The second, a study of more than three hundred cancer patients, failed to find a relation between psychosocial factors and progression of the disease.

If positive thinking has a role in the management of diseases, it is probably during the years before illness occurs. Those people who abuse themselves with fatty diets, cigarettes, alcohol and dangerous life-styles are virtually asking for trouble. Likewise, the diabetic who ignores diet, the hypertensive who disdains medicine, the heart-disease victim who does not alter his orientation, are going to regret their destructive decisions. Yet denial is unquestionably a powerful mental defense against unpleasant reality.

Dr. Marcia Angell, in a *New England Journal of Medicine* editorial, laments: "It is time to acknowledge that our belief in disease as a direct reflection of mental state is largely folklore.

Furthermore, the corollary view of sickness and death as a personal failure is a particularly unfortunate form of blaming the victim... at a time when patients are already burdened by disease...."

I think that the psyche is an important constituent of disease prevention. It permits us to adopt healthful life-styles in attempting to avoid difficulty, rather than magically altering reality once disease has developed. With all due respect to the publishing industry and TV talk shows, prevention is really where attitude counts. Self-treatment of disease by laughter and relaxation seems a more appropriate option before illness than after.

FITNESS AND GOOD HEALTH ARE NOT SYNONYMOUS

George Polk was a forty-nine-year-old postal worker who avoided cigarettes, trained regularly, was a veteran of five years of running and entered the New York City Marathon. A few weeks before the race, he dropped dead of a heart attack.

A New York City psychologist, in his late forties, jogged regularly. He had stress testing and was pronounced fit. Within a week, he collapsed in his office and died of a coronary occlusion. An autopsy revealed 60 to 90 percent blockage of his coronary arteries.

A middle-aged man who had run regularly for thirty years fought chest pain for nine miles during the New York Marathon. Halfway through the race, he suffered a major heart attack. Fortunately, he survived.

Maryland Congressman Goodloe Byron was a veteran marathoner who had completed the Boston seven times when, during a twelve-mile run in 1978, he died from a heart attack. Byron knew he had heart disease but had chosen to "run away from heart trouble," as an article in *Physician and Sportsmedicine* memorably phrased it. He repeatedly ignored cardiologists' advice to stop running. His mother had suffered angina pectoris for many years; three brothers had developed heart disease at young ages.

These examples—and others—of athletes who have suffered heart attacks while running constitute strong evidence that sports training is no guarantee of longevity.

Americans have been involved for some time now in a nationwide craze: keeping fit. Despite pronouncements by physician-joggers who claim that heart attacks and coronary arteriosclerosis are unheard of in long-distance runners, the evidence suggests that regular exercise does not protect against heart disease. In particular, runners may nurse the incorrect belief that training can produce an immunity to heart attacks. This frame of mind can cause middle-aged and older athletes to ignore warning signs like chest pain, nausea and cold sweats that may appear during exercise. In addition, current methods of evaluating athletes are not 100 percent accurate in discovering heart disease. Persons can have heart attacks during or after apparently normal exercise-cardiogram tests. Furthermore, heart attacks can occur in apparently healthy individuals *without any evidence of heart disease*. This rare event is presumably due to spasm of the arteries feeding oxygen to the heart muscle.

The benefits of regular, vigorous exercise are measurable and definable: slower pulse, lower blood pressure, reduction of blood cholesterol, improved anaerobic (low-oxygen) muscle function, improved lung function, weight loss, relief of anxiety and depression, and—perhaps most important—a pleasurable sensation and feeling of well-being.

People tend to get into trouble when, expecting too much from themselves, they exceed their physical capabilities. A prospective athlete should be aware that fitness and good health are not synonymous and should ask himself some fundamental questions: Why do I want to keep fit? So what if I am fit? Will that mean I can approach my job more effectively? Will I feel better? What are the trade-offs?

Although the quasi-religious quality of exercise worship seems to have captured the souls of millions of citizens, strenuous physical activity is certainly not a panacea for the problems of a sedentary, cigarette-smoking, alcohol- and/or Valium-dependent, obese, bored, materialistic society. As one who exercises regularly, I can testify about the enormous benefits of athletic endeavor. However, we must be cautious about attributing unrealistic consequences to fitness training. Those people who devote their lives to exercise in vain attempts to achieve the closest thing to immortality may be in for a shock. Others who exercise to feel good seem to have valid reasons for doing so. But you don't have to knock yourself out to feel good. Some heart specialists have promoted brisk walking as a reasonable middle ground between overstrenuousness and unhealthy inactivity. Such walking, for at least one hour five days a week, provides the same metabolic benefits, without risk, as an average jogging program. In other words, you don't have to be a marathoner to enjoy the blessings of regular activity.

Until recently, there were no sensible guidelines to indicate how much activity would be appropriate for a modest training program. Now exercise physiologists have developed a simple formula to enable a sportsman to estimate when he has passed from simple exertion into training. In order for an athlete to achieve *minimal* training effect, he must, at least three times a week, increase his pulse rate for five minutes to the following level: 80 percent of 220 minus his age. A twenty-year-old person must develop a pulse of 160 (220 $- 20 \times .80$); a fifty-year-old individual must exercise for five minutes with a pulse of 136 (220 $- 50 \times .80$).

Early in an exercise program, the pulse rises quickly. Therefore, the level of activity will be far lower than if a regular exerciser were to exert himself to achieve the same pulse rate. Try it. The first time you climb a steep flight of stairs or take a few hesitant jogging steps, your pulse will shoot up. After several days of this activity, your body will become accustomed to the exertion, and to achieve the same pulse rise, you will have to climb farther or run faster. In this way you can literally pace yourself. All you need is a clock and the ability to take your own pulse.

The formula is neat and quick to figure out. And it works. Your next step is to get out the skates, running shoes or cross-country skis. Welcome to the world of feeling good again.

P.S. Cigarettes don't help.

SOCIAL DRINKING

❖

Eighty years ago, regular strenuous exercise (except among the aristocracy and the poor) was not generally endorsed. Smoking was fashionable. People ate diets high in cholesterol-laden animal fat. They drank considerable amounts of alcohol.

Today we are reversing some of these trends. Exercise has become a national mania. Fewer adults are smoking cigarettes. We eat more grains and vegetables and have substantially reduced our intake of saturated fats. We no longer wish to ingest unnecessary chemicals that can harm us. Decent food, uncontaminated by the drug industry, and potable water are becoming our right, on a par with public education and voting enfranchisement. Unfortunately, we continue to consume alcohol in prodigious quantities. Americans guzzle 300 million gallons of booze a year, averaging three drinks a day for 110 million imbibers. While we cluck our tongues and shake our heads every time we read that alcoholism is an epidemic, we are positively smug in our belief that "social drinking" is a normal pattern in the fabric of our society. This belief may add to the problem, and that problem may reflect a generally abysmal ignorance about the consequences of long-term "moderate" drinking.

True, we have altered our preferences in beverages (less hard liquor, more wine), but on a per-capita basis, we consume more than we did twenty, forty, sixty years ago. Surveys indicate that 38 million drinkers ingest four or more cocktails a day, an amount proved to cause liver disease. You may be surprised to learn that alcohol-induced injury can be produced by an average daily intake of 150 grams, an amount exceeded by many social drinkers.

Few of us, physicians included, appreciate the quantity of alcohol in an ordinary drink. The following calculations, which assume a measured amount in each cocktail—and many moderate drinkers don't bother to measure—may interest you:

> Hard liquor is about 45 percent alcohol, so 100 cc. (3 ounces) contains 45 grams. Most wine is about 12.5 percent; thus a 25-ounce bottle contains 100 grams of alcohol. A six-pack of 5-percent beer provides 120 grams of alcohol.

These data cast considerable doubt on the safety of social drinking. The executive who enjoys a martini at lunch, two stiff Scotches in the evening and a glass of wine at dinner may be not only approaching but exceeding a toxic level. Social drinking is far from harmless.

In some studies, cirrhosis has been found to occur with alcohol intake as low as 20 grams (1½ drinks) a day. The four-drink-a-day consumer is six times more likely to develop cirrhosis than is a person who drinks one cocktail or less a day.

The effects of chronic alcohol abuse can be observed in almost any of the body's organs. To the liver falls the job of detoxifying alcohol, so it is considered to be a target organ. However, alcohol also causes intestinal irritation, ulcers, impaired absorption of vitamins, inflammation of the pancreas and stomach, cancer of the upper intestinal tract and liver, high blood pressure, muscle weakness, deterioration of heart muscle, reduction in male sexual ability, destruction of brain cells, mental defects resembling senility and considerable danger to the unborn children of pregnant women. All these effects have been reported in the range of what is considered by many to be "social" drinking.

On a more practical level, 3 to 5 ounces of liquor (or the equivalent in wine or beer) consumed within an hour result in serious impairment of automobile driving skills. You do not have to be drunk to have a blood level of 0.1 and be arrested for driving while intoxicated.

As in the case of cigarettes, prudence dictates that we take a hard look at what commonly available substances do to our bodies. Alcohol is fundamentally a poisonous chemical (the "toxic" in "intoxicated" *means* poison). In small quantities (less than 2 ounces a day) it is probably not harmful except to certain susceptible individuals. At quantities exceeding 6 to 8 ounces, the trouble begins. And that trouble may eventually involve more than you bargain for: the police, the hospital and the medical profession.

Most of us are familiar with the concern caused by the presence of substances like saccharin and aspartame in our diets. Diet sodas, for example, carry warnings that "this beverage may be harmful to health" because it contains one of these sugar substitutes. Years ago, some studies reportedly showed bladder cancer in rodents that were fed saccharin. If you examine the data in the reports, you will be struck by the amount of saccharin the poor mice were force-fed. The quantities were enormous and far exceeded the level any person could consume, even if he were to drink several six-packs of diet soda a day. However, soft-drink companies were required by law to inform the public of this unlikely health hazard.

So far so good. But what happened to alcoholic beverages? I don't see any disclaimers on liquor bottles or beer cans. In spite of the perfectly valid observations that juvenile drinking is a health menace and that alcoholism itself is a national epidemic, our efforts to educate ourselves continue to fail.

We have "happy hours." When it's time to "relax," we reach for a beer or two, not a good book or a chess set. The wine industry, both here and abroad, is a multibillion-dollar business, complete with its own quasi-religious rituals involving tasters and connoisseurs. In slick magazine advertisements, the beautiful people show us that to be in style and successful, we have to drink the right Scotch. About the only useful information on booze bottles describes the contents: V.S.O.P., aged 12 years, estate bottled, premium brew.

Once upon a time, cigarettes were considered adjuvants to good health. Fortunately, the incidence of smoking, at least in the adult population, is declining annually. I believe this to be an honest reflection of the thinking public's awareness of tobacco's effects. After years of trying, like all the king's men, to put smokers (with everything from emphysema to lung cancer, among other afflictions) together again, doctors began educating the public about the dangers of cigarettes. These efforts finally seem to be paying dividends.

Perhaps the moment is ripe to turn our attention to intoxicants. If I'm going to be warned about the risks of consuming an occasional diet soda, I sure as heck have a right to hear some sort of warning from brewers, distillers and wine merchants.

If disclaimers help, I'm all for them. I suggest the following information be printed on every alcohol-beverage container: "Warning: This beverage contains alcohol, an addictive and dangerous substance that can result in physical disability, brain deterioration and death." Now, that tells it like it is.

The next logical step would be to require wine and liquor manufacturers to list ingredients. That way we could discover not only the consequences of alcohol consumption but also the various goodies that are added to the brew. Liquor lobby, watch out!

DANGEROUS
DIETS

❖

In medicine, all too often the less known about the answer to a problem, the more we see written about it. Early doctors composed tomes of erudite papers about infantile paralysis, quinsy sore throat and consumption. Learned men blamed the eating of snow, bad nutrition and foul air, respectively, for these diseases. Now we recongize that the causes are poliomyelitis virus, streptococcal germs and tuberculosis bacteria. As disease becomes better understood, treatment evolves into simpler methods: vaccine for prevention of polio, penicillin for tonsillar abscess and various drugs for TB.

The modern world suffers from its own twentieth-century plagues, including cancer, arteriosclerosis and obesity. The medical literature is replete with articles by learned men who blame these diseases on a variety of causes. Treatment, like that of tuberculosis years ago, is inadequate, by and large, because the cause of each of these diseases is not understood. Take obesity, for example.

If the cause of human fatness were clearly known, we would not need the Atkins Diet, the Drinking Man's Diet, the Scarsdale Diet or any of the other fashionable diets to lose weight. Make no mistake, we are a nation of fatties. And it's not just us. The civilized world as a whole is overweight. Choose a skinny African or Asian, transplant him to the West where he can eat Twinkies and you get instant fatness.

Of course I'm speaking in hyperbole. Not all undernourished people will become obese on a Western diet, nor will all Westerners get fat on spaghetti and chocolate pudding. However, the tendency is certainly there. And it is very easy to assume the "obvious"; namely, that we are eating too many calories for our sedentary lives. Be that as it may, obesity is as typically American as ... well ... apple pie. Many overweight persons desperately try various quick ways to lose weight. Unfortunately, there are often serious consequences to these easy ways of shedding pounds.

Many popular diets, if stringently followed, result in dangerous acidosis or in nutritional deficiencies. The most disastrous consequences appear to have resulted from the liquid protein diet. So far, forty-six deaths have been attributed to this fad method of weight reduction. Here is clearly a therapeutic modality that has "outstripped its research base." Put simply, the liquid protein diet kills people because, although widely available, it has not been adequately studied.

The technique is fairly straightforward. Those unfortunate individuals who choose the liquid protein ("last chance") diet must adhere to a strict dietary intake of semisynthetic liquid protein alternating with periods of fasting. The diet certainly produces weight loss. However, when used for several months, it may also produce an irregular and inefficient heart action called "ventricular fibrillation." The heart virtually stops beating. This seems to be an unacceptable "complication" in normal patients who are, except for obesity, healthy. A leading nutritionist, Dr. Theodore Van Itallie, concluded: "... it is simply not possible to ignore the growing indication that prolonged use of the liquid protein diet is hazardous and potentially lethal. Its use in the treatment of obesity cannot be justified."

I believe we are in need of a rational approach to the problem of obesity. Prescribing diet pills, in my opinion, constitutes a malignant form of malpractice. Popular diets that allow people to eat only limited quantities of selected foods are irrational — patients won't stick to them. Liquid food substitutes produce glaring problems.

In the final analysis, obesity seems to be caused by excess calorie consumption. Although an occasional massively fat patient needs evaluation and treatment in a specialized medical center, most people who are simply overweight can easily lose pounds by avoiding foods that are rich in "empty calories." These include alcohol, processed, high-carbohydrate junk food and sugar. We seem to be consuming food that is calculated to make us fat. We could certainly profit by a return to natural, fresh vegetables and fruit and nonsynthetic protein. Maybe that's too much to ask. But it's worth thinking about. We have a lot to gain as well as much (weight) to lose.

BUNNIES AND BREAK-THROUGHS

❖

We are joined, as the saying goes, in a life-and-death battle with arteriosclerosis. As a society, we are trying desperately to find The Answer to hardening of the arteries. Before you remark that slowing the aging process is akin to discovering The Fountain of Youth (ain't been found yet) or turning lead into gold (has been done in a cyclotron), let me remind you that we think we know a little about the reasons our arterial pipes become plugged. High-cholesterol diets, cigarette smoking, excessive alcohol intake, sedentary living, genetic factors and constant exposure to stress are the current favorites.

Lest you think that doctors spend all their time in sparkling laboratories assessing the risks of Mazola versus butter in causing heart attacks, let me report that some specialists are engaged in far more serious investigational pursuits. There appears to be no limit to the extent researchers will push themselves to discover the Cause of Heart Disease. Let me explain the latest medical breakthrough.

Domestic rabbits are friendly, sweet, soft, familiar little creatures that make wonderful pets, deliver Easter eggs, have simple dietary preferences, reproduce with abandon and are legendary good friends to gentle children. Bunnies have wiggly noses, velvety paws, cute fluffy tails... and a tendency to develop massive amounts of arteriosclerosis when fed cholesterol-rich diets. The latter characteristic makes them ideal animals for use in studying hardening of the arteries.

Because of an investigation reported in the periodical *Science*, the rabbit has been immortalized. In the study group, some rabbits were petted and handled; others were not. When the rabbits were eventually autopsied, the researchers knew they were on to something big. The petted and cuddled animals showed only 40 percent of the cholesterol deposits of the control group (the uncuddled ones), even though in terms of diet, blood cholesterol, heart rates and blood pressure, the two groups were identical. It is of interest that the rabbits were all male; the handler, female.

What can one make of this? The obvious conclusion is that rabbits that are petted, held, talked to and played with on a regular basis have less arteriosclerosis than rabbits that are less fortunate. So, if you happen to be a concerned rabbit mother, these activities will help your litter to enjoy long lives. But wait! Since bunnies tend to follow the human pattern with respect to heart disease, surely some conclusion can be made about people. You can bet that it was. The authors concluded that since petting protected the rabbits, it should also protect humans. I exaggerate but, believe me, I know what was going through those doctors' minds. They could smell a Nobel prize.

If we can believe the bunny study, humans who are played with and loved would fare better than those who are not. You may be able to eat eggs Benedict with impunity, smoke to your heart's content, drink like a fish, cease all strenuous exercise, forget your genes and thoroughly enjoy a frustrating life of anxiety—in other words, be a normal American—if only you are petted and cuddled. I don't know about you, but I think this is the best news since Dorothy clicked her heels together and got back to Kansas.

I am not suggesting you go out and find a New Bunny to take care of you. However, getting snuggled certainly beats giving up Scotch and chocolate mousse. At last I understand why certain strangely sexist men sport little black-and-white logos of a rabbit head. All this time I thought these would-be playboys were proclaiming that they were swingers. Now I can fully appreciate that these bunny worshipers are really at the forefront of medical knowledge. They are effectively expressing their support of a life-style calculated to reduce hardening of the arteries. *Playboy* magazine must be to cardiologists what *Sunshine and Health* is to dermatologists: just another medical journal.

IT DOESN'T ALWAYS HAPPEN TO THE OTHER GUY

❖

About five years ago, a television commercial extolling the virtues of Lifesaver candies embodied an approach to life and health I find disquieting. The spoken message told us that each Lifesaver contains *only* ten calories, so enjoy a handful. The insidious unspoken message is: "Look, sure you're fat and shouldn't eat candy, but what's a lousy ten calories going to matter? Give in to temptation and deal later with the consequences."

We all know people who are careful and conscientious about their health and well-being, sometimes to an extreme degree. Here I am talking about those who tend to defer responsibility for themselves, an attitude that can reflect the mouth-watering successes of contemporary medical treatment. Years ago, there seemed to be a clear relation between action and reaction. Today, that relation has become blurred. Many consumers seem willing, almost eager, to bargain with reality. Let me explain.

A century ago, if a house was quarantined and you entered it, you knew you would be exposed to a dread disease, probably contract it and have to deal with the results, which in cases of typhoid fever and bubonic plague usually meant death. If you chose to travel to the tropics, you were very likely to come down with malaria—and that was that; you either died or put up with a cyclic, untreatable disease. In the past, venereal disease was an extremely uncomfortable and incurable affliction that lead to sterility, dementia or death. There was very little doubt how you got it; you paid your figurative (or literal) money and took your chances.

Modern medicine has, happily, changed situations like these for the better. Yet there has been an unexpected trade-off. True, we've found cures for many diseases—but have we lost something important along the way? Are we now fooling ourselves into believing we can postpone responsibility, hoping we can cheat fate?

Adolescents do this best because they believe that accidents and serious diseases *always* happen to someone else, usually a faceless, far-off, unknown victim. The average young adult views himself as invulnerable. We tend to carry this fantasy into middle age. I am convinced that the aging and maturing process carries with it the depressing realization that bad things do happen to many people and these people are folks we know, have grown up and worked with, said hello to, cared about, loved, parented. As we get old we begin to appreciate just how tenuous life is and that bad things, horror of horrors, can happen even to us . . . and do so with increasing frequency as we age.

Unfortunately, the successful medical treatment we're becoming accustomed to seduces many of us into behaving as though we need not take responsible action in the present; we can afford to wait until later. Smoke cigarettes, eat and drink excessively, drive carelessly, mistreat ourselves—we can always pay the piper later, or, if treatment works, perhaps never.

I wish more people appreciated how desperately inadequate doctors really are. Certainly, we can accomplish wonders, but, ultimately, we are limited simply to helping people help themselves. This arrangement is painfully obvious to adults as they grow older, but it seems inane to the young.

If the term "preventive medicine" has relevance, it is this: starting in childhood, each person has the potential of taking a series of actions to protect health. That responsibility does not begin after forty. By then, it may be too late.

CHAPTER 9

BODY
AND
SOUL

RUNNING
AMOK

❖

In college, I majored in sociology. The study of societies was a fascinating introduction to the ways in which people of the world deal with problems threatening their existences as tribes and civilizations. Then I moved into psychology, which studies the ways individuals deal with personal, internal problems. Eventually, I chose a career in medicine, which, I suppose, addresses how we deal with more individual, still smaller-scale problems involving tissues and organs.

Despite what might be called a "refinement of discipline," I am still a student of sociology. And to this day, I am tantalized by the medical aspects of that subject. Take, for example, the concept of *heva*, an obscure behavioral condition observed only among inhabitants of Easter Island. Once a person has been told his kinsman was murdered, he may develop *heva* by seizing a live rat in his mouth and charging around the neighborhood with a huge club, making mayhem and seeking revenge.

This pattern is somewhat similar to a phenomenon called *amok*, which is indigenous to Malaysia. After experiencing profound depression, a man may erupt into a temporary state of violent frenzy during which he homicidally attacks other people around him. If he is not himself killed in turn, he may experience amnesia. Unfortunately, the patient with *amok* is now likely to be a police problem, even in "civilized" countries. Witness the lurid newspaper reports that describe in gory detail how snipers hole up in towers and pop away at pedestrians or how supposedly normal family men go berserk and attempt, sometimes successfully, to slaughter family, friends, and neighbors.

Less serious, but no less interesting, is the syndrome of *latah* in South Asia. The victim, usually a middle-aged woman of low social status, responds to sudden loud noises or tickling by a total loss of self-control. She may scream, become hysterical, involuntarily utter obscenities, drop objects, and obey the commands or mimic the words of observers. This uncontrollable startle reaction has been reported in other countries as "The Jumping Frenchman of Maine," "Lapp Panic" in England and *ikota* in Siberia. No one understands why it occurs. One might justifiably inquire what survival function is served by *heva, amok* and *latah*. I don't know.

Koro is another form of bizarre orientation confined, fortunately, to Southeast Asia. The apprehensive sufferer of this malady becomes convinced that his penis is shrinking and will eventually recede into his belly and that death will ensue. Although women may experience *koro* as the disappearance of their breasts and labia, it is men (in these characteristically sexist societies) who try to prevent its consequences. They use penile expanders or firmly grasp and stretch their organs in vain attempts to prevent the poor things from retracting. They often enlist the help of other people to serve this function. In fact, no *koro* victim has ever died of the condition, but many are said to be brain-damaged or intoxicated with alcohol and other drugs when the fit takes them.

While we may be alternately shocked and amused by these abberations, they are real phenomena within each culture. Modern anthropologists are equally interested in stress-provoked reactions characteristic of the Western world. Is our current compulsion to stockpile nuclear weapons a sophisticated example of *heva*? Are the so-called "developed countries" running *amok*?

The next time you see your doctor running through town in a frenzy, gripping a live rat in his mouth, brandishing an eight-inch butcher knife, muttering obscenities, and clutching his groin, please be understanding. We too have tensions and try to express them in socially acceptable ways.

DOES WITCH-DOCTORING WORK?

The African witch doctor is now termed a "practitioner of traditional medicine." I suppose that makes me a practitioner of radical medicine, a hard label for me to endure... but that's beside the point.

Witch doctors use many interesting methods to diagnose disease. They throw sticks and examine the patterns. They study the configurations of dry chicken bones. They shake seeds in a gourd; depending on how the seeds pour out of the gourd, the witch doctor can verify the cause of a certain malady. The basis of illness runs the gamut from intricate enchantments to something as mundane as the patient having forgotten to give a chicken to his in-laws.

Before your slap your thigh and giggle, consider that the gourd approach, for example, may not be as bizarre as it sounds.

To begin with, there is the element of chance. No one, presumably, knows the exact sequence in which the seeds fall from the gourd. Since most people recover from illness, what is the difference if the cause is streptococcus, anxiety depression or one chicken too many? Even modern Western doctors play a game of chance, which we call statistics. Aunt Margaret is critically ill. Here are the lab results (seeds); let's try this new medicine and see if it works.

In the second place, witch doctors avoid placing obstacles in the way of their patients' recovery. Isn't it much easier to give away a domestic animal—and recover one's health—than to stop smoking? Or cut out the martini at lunch? Or eat less?

Finally, witch doctors involve their patients in treatment. If a patient (or his relative) *does* something, a cure may be forthcoming. This is a radical departure from so-called modern medicine, in which the patient has little to say about treatment, loses control and is basically at the mercy of his doctor.

You see, if you believe a certain factor—any factor—is the cause of your discomfort, its removal or modification may be curative, even if that factor is not really to blame. A twentieth-century housewife is told that her headache is due to tension and she had better stop worrying about whether her youngster makes the Pee-Wee hockey team. An African woman is told that the cause of her headache is that she didn't stay long enough in the jungle during her menstruation. Each woman takes the advice offered by her practitioner and improves. Which doctor is the witch doctor?

Obviously, primitive medicine men operate at a tremendous disadvantage in dealing with diseases such as infections and cancer. Nonetheless, modern doctors could learn a lot from them with respect to bedside manners and "psychosomatic" conditions. My opposite number in Kenya unfortunately shares my prejudice; we are suspicious of each other.

Here is where the scientific method comes in so handy. It enables an unbiased third party to make an objective judgment about diagnosis and treatment. On the basis of this method, we are able to conclude that a certain root, a form of faith healing or a brand of psychosurgery is not effective. The constant testing of civilized medicine is crucial to its success, as testing is mandatory to the success of any intellectual system. Fortunately, Western-trained African doctors are now seriously investigating Third World traditional medicine in order to discover which, if any, techniques and medicines might be beneficial to the world community. Inasmuch as many discoveries have been based on primitive folklore—the development of curare, digitalis and antibiotics, for example—there is much potential information to be gained from the study of "traditional" medicine in any society. Perhaps a cancer cure lies hidden away in the Amazon jungle.

All this talk of science is fine. However, in my heart of hearts I have known all along that the true basis of my problem is simple: I cannot bring myself to give an extra goat to my wife's family.

MAL
IN ANY
LANGUAGE

❖

Those of us who practice medicine in the so-called developed world make certain assumptions that are considered by people in other countries to be ludicrous. In most "undeveloped" nations, illness is an extremely private matter. Healers' efforts to discover the causes of disease are viewed as invasions. Therefore, these efforts are perceived as more than ineffectual; they can be downright dangerous. No wonder some Third World patients adopt attitudes of secrecy and lament that Western doctors don't "understand" illness.

For example, the Quechua Indians, in the Central Andes of Peru, have developed a complex system of medical care that is based on the guinea pig, or *cuy*.

In the Quechuan civilization, *mal* is one of life's inevitabilities. Loosely translated, *mal* means a combination of sickness, evil and envy. When *mal* enters the body, the patient becomes diseased. Treatment with modern medicine may temporarily alleviate symptoms, but unless *mal* is removed, the patient cannot be cured.

The *cuy* is used to remove *mal*. The healer takes a guinea pig and performs a ritual called *radiografia con el cuy*, which involves massaging the patient's body with corresponding body parts of the live guinea pig. After the *cuy* absorbs *mal*, it is cut open and examined. Analysis of the animal's innards enables the healer to document and define the nature of the patient's illness.

A good native healer recognizes more than just *mal*; he or she must be able to identify in what ways human sickness is reflected in the *cuy*. Then the offending parts of the animal must be appropriately buried. In essence, disease is not simply eliminated in humans; it is transferred to the guinea pig and then disposed of.

For his part, the healer is always evasive and never gives useful information when questioned because to do so would enable an envious person to cast a spell and cause disease in someone else. The healer is versed in recognizing the fundamental essence of illness; the patient may be totally unaware of its manifestations.

Although Peruvian folk medicine may seem obscenely primitive to us self-proclaimed sophisticates, the Indians, after being treated by Western doctors, will go elsewhere to be healed. Their medical system is based on a set of beliefs that predate the Spanish Conquest. Compared to them, we are newcomers. You have to give them credit for such loyalty. The whole arrangement makes you appreciate the importance of Believing as an integral part of Healing.

Come to think of it, our viewpoints are not that dissimilar. U.S. doctors view disease as an imbalance of forces within the body. That is, cancer cells or depressing brain chemicals or virulent microorganisms or toxins of one kind or another—in a word, *mal*—are in the body. These substances or agents must be neutralized or destroyed. In this effort, doctors talk in magical languages and rarely choose to provide useful information to the patient or the family. We are evasive. By our own admission, we do not understand the basis, the real basis, of disease.

What really causes heart attacks? Well, they might be the result of blood clots caused by *mal*. Cancer is certainly *mal* in any language. Why are some people with gallstones able to eat greasy cheeseburgers while others roll on the floor after consuming fettucini? Nobody knows. Maybe it's *mal*. Do we need to change our orientation and begin to examine our patients' spiritual health as well as their bodies? Perhaps the root of disease does, after all, lie in the soul.

I, for one, might sometimes vote for *cuys* over chemotherapy; guinea pig cures are safer, and the Peruvians seem to be content to address the patient as a whole, rather than as a collection of isolated parts. If the university hospital ever develops a Department of Guinea Pig Medicine and is looking for a chairman, I would be tempted to be among the first in line to interview for the job.

SPRAYING EVIL AWAY

❖

Several reports concerning health problems of the underprivileged have appeared in the medical literature. One of the most interesting, "Folk Medical Beliefs and Their Implications for Care of Patients," was published in the *Annals of Internal Medicine* some ten years ago. The authors' conclusions, which I feel are still valid today, were based on an in-depth study of a poor black community in Tucson, Arizona. However, judging from a list of 112 additional studies cited in the report, the beliefs were comparable to those already recognized among underprivileged Mexican-Americans, Puerto Rican–Americans and southern whites. The implication is that unless doctors are aware of certain folk beliefs—many of which are at odds with scientific medicine—we may be less effective at times than we might be in dealing with medical problems of the disadvantaged.

Some illness was seen as reflecting malice from an evildoer, God, evil spirits or opposing external forces. This type of "natural illness" is described as being very real to the people in the communities studied, and the article points out that patients who believe themselves affected by such "magical" diseases rarely seek medical help from qualified physicians. Rather, they would prefer to see folk healers. Or they might attempt self-cure with commercially available charms and magical means. "Oils, incenses, candles, and aerosol room sprays may be used to repel evil."

When I read this article, in an interested but detached frame of mind, I stored the information away in the category of "worth-

while but not immediately useful." A few hours later, while
watching television, I was amused to see an advertisement about
Lysol spray. Obviously beamed to a middle-class audience, the
ad showed a woman and her child entering a public restroom.
She had her trusty Lysol, which, she happily indicated, she
would use to spray the toilet seat to kill "germs" left by other
people.

To me, the message was unmistakable. Here was Madison
Avenue flagrantly appealing to a superstition that, although generally considered to be representative of the uneducated, may
actually affect us all. The advertising industry has led us to
believe that ever-present "germs" are swarming to do us harm.
Billions of little green, vibrating, bug-eyed menaces are bump-
ing together like pond-water algae, with suckers or hooks, crazed,
with their only goal in life to infect human beings from toilet
seats—or motel rooms or shower floors. I thought of the Chicanos
using aerosol sprays to repel evil, and I realized this very human
and irrational tendency is probably universal.

The all-inclusive term "bacteria" encompasses thousands of
varieties of microscopic, one-celled primitive creatures that are
present throughout our environment. From a practical standpoint, something is considered to be "sterile" when it contains
no bacteria or other microorganisms (fungus, yeasts and so forth).

In the human body, any surface exposed to the air has bacteria on it. These surfaces include skin, hair, mouth, lungs and
the gastrointestinal tract. Normally, internal "surfaces"—like
the bloodstream, muscles, bones, joints, brain, nerves and the
upper genitourinary system—are free of bacteria.

In our environment, bacteria are ubiquitous. They are present everywhere: in air, soil and water. Most bacteria are entirely
innocuous; they do no harm and are actually necessary in the
normal chain of nature. For example, bacteria around plant roots
produce nitrogen that is necessary for growth. Some animals—
like grass-eating mammals—require bacteria in their intestines
in order to manufacture certain vitamins.

All in all, living creatures have a very satisfactory relationship with their bacteria. Over the millennia, a balance between

nonpathogenic (harmless) bacteria and their hosts has been established. Nevertheless, nature is predictably unkind.

There is a small group of bacteria that are harmful (pathogenic) to their hosts. This group includes species of organisms that scientists have classed as disease causers: strep, staph, pneumococci and the types of bacteria that produce diphtheria, tuberculosis, venereal disease, typhoid and other—often fatal—illnesses in humans.

To the great credit of medical scientists, chemicals have been developed to kill these bacteria. Although most antibiotics only help a person's natural defenses by weakening pathogenic bacteria, the drugs have been of inestimable value in saving lives and reducing the discomfort of bacterial infection in millions of patients.

With people's increasing knowledge about bacteria, it was inevitable that some companies would, with success, try to play upon the fear that we have all developed about "bacterial infection." For instance, Listerine and Lysol are currently being advertised to produce "clean breath" and a clean environment, respectively, as a result of their bacteria-killing properties. While it is true that these compounds do, in fact, kill bacteria, the consumer would do well to demand more precision in evaluating their claims.

As an example, the mouth contains billions of harmless bacteria. Some forms of bad breath are caused by bacterial decomposition of food between teeth. Listerine—and many other mouthwashes—will kill millions of bacteria on contact, but only a tiny proportion of the *total*. Furthermore, as soon as the Listerine has been spit out, billions of bacteria are reintroduced into the mouth during breathing and eating. So while the consumer's mouth will feel "fresh," in fact the bacterial count rapidly rises to "pretreatment" levels; essentially, nothing has been accomplished.

Lysol spray when applied to surfaces will kill some bacteria, but most of these are nonpathogens and would do us no harm anyway. Bacteria that cause venereal disease die quickly outside the body and would be unlikely to reside on public toilet seats long enough for the spray to make any difference. The Lysol spray will scent the air, however, and that seems to be the important consideration. Somehow, if we don't see or smell the germs, we assume they're all gone. The room must be safe. The evil has been repelled. We can take a shower.

Several studies have shown that plain soap and water is a superior disinfectant. Toothbrushing certainly is more effective than mouthwashing. And if a potentially harmful infection should develop, our bodies will make it known to us through pain, fever, swelling or redness.

For those of us who rely on myriad sprays, lotions and mouthwashes, let us do so with the full realization of what they are, and are not, accomplishing—and not unfairly involve the lowly microbe.

DEATH OF THE WOLF BOY

❖

Ramu, the Wolf Boy of India, died at age ten in a home for paupers run by Mother Teresa's Missionaries of Charities. His death poses fascinating anthropological questions and raises some pertinent medical issues.

As reported in *The New York Times*, the youngster developed cramps in early February 1985 and died two weeks later, after having "failed to respond to medical treatment."

He was first discovered in 1976 living with three wolf cubs in the desolate jungle of Sultanpur. His fingernails and toenails were like claws; his elbows and knees were callused. He walked on all fours and fought against capture. He preferred to eat raw meat and would raid chicken coops near the convent where he was initially—and apparently unsuccessfully—restrained.

Zoologists attributed his survival to the wolf pack, which had treated him as one of its cubs. Because he never learned to speak—although he could bathe and dress himself—he was unable to supply the details of his early upbringing, even if he remembered them.

An astute observer of mammalian behavior might be tempted to conclude that Ramu was more animal than human. Is it possible that his infant year with the wolves so altered his development that nine years of human influence failed to transform him? Or was his desperate clinging to an animal affiliation a sad testimonial to the inadequacies of Indian institutions for the homeless?

Although materially impoverished, Ramu may in fact have been rich in a heritage that his human masters didn't want to believe or couldn't understand. He was not described as "retarded" in the classical sense. Perhaps this unique child saw both worlds and preferred the first one as the lesser of two evils.

Of course, a humanist would argue that Ramu's early deprivations forever warped his ability to be human; he may have been incalculably and indelibly injured by his feral state. Yet I think it's fair to speculate that he made an atavistic choice of sorts.

Why did he die? With all the so-called miracles of modern medicine at the disposal of the Indian doctors—and I assume they had every scientific gadget available—why were they unable to save this fierce and independent ten-year-old?

In an age characterized by the glories of electronic wizardry, Ramu surely could have been kept alive, in the Karen Ann Quinlan mode, for months or years. But he succumbed after a mere two weeks with abdominal cramps.

If we have the power to keep the terminally ill alive, what was the indefinable essence that Ramu lacked?

I believe that essence may have been the will to live, the spirit. We doctors tend to ignore characteristics that cannot be measured, quantified, recorded, plotted on a graph. But there is an unmeasurable factor in every human life that may be as important to survival as surgery and antibiotics: spirit, will—even, perhaps, soul.

Ramu's time had come, evidently. I suspect he knew it.

Perhaps his doctors—in their inscrutably unfamiliar Eastern way—knew it too. Still, it seems a shame that the boy couldn't hold on to life long enough to achieve adulthood. He must have possessed tremendous spunk to endure his first year in the wild, and then nine years in a facility for "sick and dying destitutes."

Was he sick in soul? Terminally ill from a spiritual nihilism that science is still waiting to comprehend?

No matter how charitable the institution, I wonder which one of us would choose to exist indefinitely among dying destitutes. What did the Wolf Boy require that he wasn't given? Are not the intangible needs of sick and emotionally bankrupt patients in our own society often ignored?

Ramu deserves credit for living, both in and out of captivity, as long as he did. Perhaps his experience will provide a basis for re-evaluation of the ways we view and treat disease, because intravenous feedings, dialysis, respirators and pacemakers aren't enough. Are they?

CHAPTER 10

BUCKSHOT

BIG
PEEVES
IN
SMALL
PACKAGES

❖

You would think that with all the technological skills at our disposal, someone could invent a workable pipe reamer.

For those of you who don't smoke pipes, I allude to the chore that we pipe smokers periodically confront: cleaning out the charred ash that forms inside the pipe bowl. The stuff is abominable. It's as hard as dried plastic wood. It builds up, smoke after smoke, like malignant arteriosclerosis, progressively reducing the diameter of the bowl until so little tobacco can be inserted that a relaxing after-dinner habit becomes a five-minute frustration.

Of more economic importance, the gummy crust has a different coefficient of expansion than does wood. If the pipe is not regularly reamed—a major undertaking, at present—the briar expands at a different rate than the deposit and will crack, thereby ruining the pipe.

I realize that this is not the kind of technological problem that interests the general public. Perhaps it is an inconvenience better suited to analysis by Andy Rooney. However, I have yet to find a decent, cleanable, inexpensive pipe reamer. And that got me thinking about other familiar items that could stand some improvement.

• The stethoscope. Contrary to popular belief, physicians do not store their stethoscopes in the coldest crannies of the office. In fact, I often warm the flat, listening portion, called the diaphragm, before placing it on an unsuspecting warm chest. But the warming is never enough. Each patient jumps up and exclaims: "Hey, Doc, where do you keep that thing? [You guessed the next line.] In the refrigerator?"

I plead for someone to design a stethoscope mitten—or

something—so that doctors can stop torturing warm-blooded clients.

• The hospital gown. This flimsy cotton garment was clearly not designed by a patient for a patient. The darned thing is a veritable Gordian knot of flaps, snaps, ties and gaping holes. I've never met a patient who could figure out how to get into it. Never met a doctor who could, either. If you slip it on with the opening in the front—the logical way—watch out: you end up looking like a refugee from *Penthouse* magazine. When donned with the opening in the back, the gown exposes the entire spinal column, down to and including the coccyx and surrounding structures.

This vestment defies my definition of the word "gown." It seems calculated to minimize modesty, maximize loss of body heat and make the wearer an instant object of interest to visitors. I say throw hospital gowns into the wastebasket and insist on wearing your pajamas or nighties. (Incidentally, the disposable office gown is no improvement over its hospital counterpart.)

• Stirrups. These are not the gadgets you stuff your boots into when cantering around the countryside. Medical stirrups are medieval devices—akin to the thumbscrew—commonly attached to uncomfortable tables upon which sadistic gynecologists examine women's reproductive tracts. The specialists insist that stirrups are necessary, but most females don't like them, and I've never seen a male gynecologist try them himself. The solution? Ride bareback. Or surprise your obstetrician by requesting a western saddle.

• Tongue depressors. These ubiquitous, rounded flat wooden blades have probably been used since Cro-Magnon times for looking into throats. They never fail to make their victims gag. Their sole value, it seems to me, is to provide a surface upon which pediatricians can draw little faces so children can take them home, break them, get splinters and return to the doctor.

The secret? Don't stick your tongue out if you're examined with a tongue blade; the nerves that trigger the gag reflex live contentedly in the back of the tongue. Either allow the doctor to use a tongue depressor or stick your tongue out, not both.

Although modern science can put men and women in space, I suspect that what we really need are more enterprising young minds devoted to discovering solutions to our little problems. One way or the other, the big ones have a tendency to take care of themselves.

GENERIC DOCTORING

❖

Clearly, many Americans are becoming extremely cost-conscious. In the process, they are also becoming less discriminating. This phenomenon has resulted in the supermarket boom called generic buying, which has now been extended to bulk generic buying. No longer content with purchasing Basic toilet paper and light bulbs, housewives are dipping into plastic cracker barrels for pancake mix, pasta, bread flour, pie filling mix and spices.

What used to be called patients (but are now known as Consumers of Health Services) seem increasingly more inclined to visit non-office-based physicians: the generic equivalent, if you will, of the family doctor, who at least had a name.

If people want to see a doctor and they do not choose to wait for an appointment, they line up at the hospital emergency room or go to the newest-of-the-new gimmicks, Doc-in-the-Box, a strictly daytime facility that caters to walk-ins—but not after hours, please. This is true generic buying. Although emergency room physicians are generally well trained, they are fundamentally a no-name product and—paradoxically—more expensive than their office counterparts. Further, they are far removed from the unsubsidized family doctor whose strengths, weaknesses, quirks and level of training are recognized by his patients. Because about 50 percent of emergency room visits are not emergencies at all, I am intrigued by the ways this patient glut must reduce the standard of care necessary for handling true emergency cases.

I am also intrigued by an apparent contradiction. I've heard tell that today's doctors exhibit many unattractive peculiarities, such as being financially oriented, unwilling to give adequate time to each patient, refusing to develop a warm doctor-patient relation: in essence, the very qualities that traditionally characterize emergency rooms.

I guess some patients are willing to forgo the human experience of letting a physician get to know them. Maybe it's safer to deal with a conveyor belt of unfamiliar M.D.s. It certainly matters a lot that insurance coverage picks up part of the tab in the hospital setting. But one fact remains clear: a patient will get the best and least expensive care from a doctor whom he knows ... and who, in turn, knows the patient, his idiosyncrasies, his medical history and the medicines he is taking. I think it makes more sense to change doctors, if that is desirable, than to go scooting off to a "generic doctor" for a cold or a backache.

For all I know, Basic beer may be manufactured by a premium brewery; No-Name paper napkins may be as good as the best; generic soda may be "the real thing." If so, the cost certainly shouldn't escalate if the words "Schlitz," "Scott" and "Coke" are added to the packages.

In a medical setting, I insist on knowing where my doctor trained, whether he is a skillful diagnostician, and if I can count on him at night and during off-hours.

You are as likely to find ants in your generic sugar as you are to find an incompetent physician working the emergency room at an accredited hospital. But the facelessness of it, the overutilization of hospital facilities, the overemphasis on machines and tests seem to me to be encouraging the very process of dehumanization we all object to in the medical profession. Any good doctor knows his patients and makes a special effort to treat the person, not just the disease. Generic buying is a device best left in the supermarket; it is more suited to commodities than to people.

BLAMING
THE
PATIENT

❖

Everybody who lives in Florida drives a white car with tinted windows.

Italians always grow grapes in their backyards.

Rather than printing the truth, editors prefer to publish sensational material that will sell newspapers, magazines and books.

All car salesmen are dishonest.

We are fascinated by stereotypes. Our lives revolve around caricatured concepts of people and groups.

Politicians can't be trusted.

All doctors are rich.

Male hairdressers are homosexual.

Many stereotypes are reassuring to the believer because he can gain a bizarre sense of superiority by pigeonholing other people. But stereotyping is demeaning to the person being stereotyped. Unfortunately, doctors, being human, are as likely to stereotype as the next fellow. This is a current favorite: patients bring illness on themselves.

Now, in many instances this is true. The heavy cigarette smoker is clearly asking for trouble with respect to emphysema and lung cancer. Those invulnerable young men who, helmetless, jockey motorcycles at high speeds on crowded thoroughfares are risking their own lives as well as the safety of other citizens. The diabetic who refuses to eat properly is inviting calamity.

However, people—perfectly normal, law-abiding people— often get sick or are injured through no fault of their own. Things just . . . happen. You develop angina or a cancer or a cold. And that's it. You didn't ask for the problem; it resulted from factors beyond your control.

Yet many doctors seem to take perverse delight in trying to

identify causes that make the patient in some way completely responsible for his own misfortune. This happens, I believe, because it enables the doctor to relinquish some of his responsibility. How comforting to know that the patient was so willful or ignorant as to bring unpleasantness on himself. The law of cause and effect is—however vaguely—reaffirmed. Blame the patient; that's far safer than admitting that we do not really know the causes of heart disease, malignancy and coryza.

I'll tell you something. I know people who don't go to doctors. And for good reason. They enjoy good health and they don't like white-coated technicians, X rays, fancy gadgets, and intimidation by overweight doctors who smoke and wouldn't dream of exposing themselves to the humiliation of a medical examination. I don't agree with these non-doctorgoers because I fancy myself a good physician and believe that we can often be indispensable when illness strikes. But, by Hippocrates, I can respect a person's reluctance to sit and listen to a doctor reel off all the reasons a patient should feel guilty for being sick. In the last analysis, we all know quite accurately what we are doing wrong to ourselves. What we need is additional knowledge and, most of all, help in coping with illness.

Ten years ago, you developed diverticulitis from eating too much roughage. Salads, vegetable fiber and "indigestible foods" were no-nos. If you got a bellyache, doctors were delighted to analyze meticulously where you went wrong. They pronounced judgment: it was the endive you ate last Wednesday.

Today the word is that roughage is *good*. You are encouraged to eat fiber. Indigestible bran is "in." Diverticulitis results from salad-poor diets. You can't win.

I think we just have to realize that piteously little is known about most diseases. Blame the Patient is a game that has to go. Moderation remains a reasonable compromise, in conjunction with periodic examinations and appropriate alertness to changes in bodily function. Less intimidation and more information would certainly make your next visit to the doctor more bearable.

FREE
ADVICE

❖

The matronly dowager drew herself up to full height and, with a conspiratorial wink, confided in a stage whisper: "What you need, my dear, is *exercise*! You must walk, walk, walk. *Force* yourself!" The words were directed at my patient, a lovely woman with angina and a weak heart. If she had walked, particularly in the cold air that day, she would have had chest pain and shortness of breath. Despite the medicine she took daily, exercise was definitely to be avoided. If she had forced herself to walk, the activity could have been downright dangerous. Although the matron was well intentioned, her advice could have had disastrous consequences.

Other examples abound. "Got a headache? Here, my doctor gave me these fabulous pills. Try one." The giver of this free advice did not reflect on the fact that headaches have different causes requiring individual treatment. In addition, suppose the recipient was allergic to a compound in the medicine or had a peculiar reaction? A simple headache could be turned into a serious medical emergency.

"Ah, you just twisted your ankle. My uncle says to use hot packs right away!" When the heat causes further bleeding into injured tissue and the ankle balloons out like a sore blue sausage, the injury victim may conclude that the "treatment" was worse than the sprain.

We all have a natural tendency to want to help a fellow human being who is experiencing discomfort. For the most part, casual advice exchanged between friends can have a beneficial effect. However, most doctors are familiar with situations in which unqualified but caring people have given opinions or advice about potentially serious situations. As public sophistication about medical subjects increases, there is a tendency for nonprofessionals to assume knowledge and make judgments that are often inappropriate.

In my opinion, good nonprofessional advice can usually be couched in fairly vague but constructive terms. Take, for example, the patient who is suffering prolonged discomfort. Rather than suggest to such a person: "These pills helped me when I was sick, so try them," a more appropriate approach might be: "I'm concerned that you're not feeling better. Why don't you talk to your doctor about it? I'm sure he wouldn't object to your getting another opinion." This sort of open-ended encouragement can do an enormous amount of good without placing upon the adviser a burden that may exceed his competence.

Conversely, the recipient would do well to take with the proverbial grain of salt any pseudotechnical pronouncements made by friends, relatives or colleagues.

Being helpful does not necessarily mean providing definitive answers to problems. It can mean pointing someone in a proper direction to find needed assistance. Although free advice seems to have become commonplace, we might remind ourselves that, as with other commodities, you get what you pay for.

HOLY MOLY! WHAT A WAY TO MAKE A BUCK!

❖

Not long ago, I received an outlandish offer in the mail. For those few of you who don't believe there is still a buck to be made in the practice of medicine, I herewith introduce you to the International Institute of Bach Practitioners. (It bears no relation to the J. S. Bach and sons who wrote music.) I am not yet a member of this august organization, which is based in Madras, India, but I have been invited to join. All I have to do is enroll

in an eighteen-month diploma course and ante up a mere $120. At the conclusion of the correspondence study, I am promised an IBP diploma that will enable me to treat the halt and the lame with Bach Flower Remedies.

In the unlikely event that you are blissfully ignorant of this miraculous medical breakthrough, the IBP defines it as "A New and Complete System of Medical Therapeutics for the cure of all diseases—physical as well as psychological—with just thirty-eight remedies prepared from Wild Flowers. These are absolutely harmless and produce NO SIDE EFFECTS! They are NON-HABITFORMING and are highly efficacious! Easy to carry, sweet in taste!!"

The head petal in this bouquet of practitioners, Dr. V. Krishnamoorty, not only wants my 120 U.S. dollars, but declares I will be able to cure all illness with just thirty-eight—count them, thirty-eight—flower compounds. Why, I ask myself, am I busting my buns learning about calcium channel blockers, third-generation cephalosporins and recombinant-DNA research when the Bach Flower Remedies are sitting in some Indian warehouse waiting to cure common ailments as well as disorders I've never heard of?

For example, Cherry Plum seems to be a real winner. It is the "remedy PAR EXCELLENCE" (according to Dr. V. Krishnamoorty) for burns, scalds, dehyration, vomiting, lacerations, "unbearable suffering" and "hopelessness." Star of Bethlehem reverses the effects of electrocution. Scleranthus relieves laziness so that patients who "have the habit of postponing things . . . and are always late in getting up from their bed" can become "alert, active and busy."

There's more. Chestnutbud counteracts slow learning. Honeysuckle enables the patient to pounce on "any golden opportunities." Crab Apple makes a short person tall, a fat person thin and anybody more physically fit; it also cures pimples and baldness. Larch increases self-confidence; Willow deflates superiority complex; Vine cures adolescence.

White Chestnut is useful for "mental derangements, u

wanted thoughts, always counting one to hundred, excessive joy
and hallucinations." Walnut "helps one to easily give up coffee,
tobacco, alcohol, etc."

Holy Moly! as Captain Marvel used to say. The whole medical
profession probably could alleviate all its own woes by using
this stuff. But I have no intention of freely giving away all Dr.
V. Krishnamoorty's glorious secrets.

The thirty-eight remedies are individually packaged in one-
ounce plastic "phials," each containing "about 600 pills." Each
phial costs $17. Each dose is two pills. Let's see ... at $10 a
dose ... that's $3,000 profit per bottle, minus $17, times thirty-
eight bottles ... I give up. The calculations are too tough, unless
I take Chestnutbud.

The whole scheme really sounds like the scam of the decade.
I'm told that if I invest $120, wait eighteen months, purchase
a closetful of premade flower extracts and adopt the Bach philosophy, I can achieve instant success. Furthermore, I will be
able to cure everything from scabies to schizophrenia. If these
claims are in doubt, I've been given the name of a Greenwich,
Connecticut, doctor as a reference.

While reading through the Bach Flower Remedy brochure,
I thanked my lucky stars for scientists of objective persuasion
who, through hard work and sacrifice, eradicated smallpox,
tamed syphilis, wiped out plague, prevented polio and generally
performed valuable services for mankind. I am saddened that
the faults and drawbacks of twentieth-century medicine force
desperate patients to seek alternative, unproved treatments. No
system is perfect. Nonetheless, despite its flaws, ours has provided the most benefits and holds more sturdy promise for the
future.

I think I'm fairly broad-minded, but Bach's remedies seem
to me to be outrageous artifices that prey on innocent, gullible
unfortunates. I reluctantly came to that conclusion after I ate
two dozen daisies, threw up all afternoon and still don't know
if she loves me or loves me not.

OF COLLY-WOBBLES AND PIDIDDLES

❖

Garbagemen are dead.

Yes, folks, there are no more garbagemen. They have been replaced by Sanitary Engineers and Refuse Specialists.

Know what? There are no more domestics. Instead we are blessed with Housekeepers. These hardy, modern womenpersons may or may not perform the work of what used to be known as housecleaners, cooks and servants—it's hard to tell because of Specialization. In today's world of strangespeak, I'm not surprised that so many domestics are foreign.

I vote for a wake and memorial service to honor janitors. These dear departed have passed on. In their places are Custodians.

There was a time in this country when a day's honest labor was regarded with respect. There was no stigma attached to manual work. A wage earner was not ashamed to be identified with steady menial effort. Today, not only is unskilled work disdained by many of the poor—now known as the disadvantaged—but we are increasingly living in a world of strangespeak. For those of you who don't know it, the state of Connecticut no longer has a welfare department. Before you begin cheering, let me add that only the name has been changed, to the Department of Income Maintenance. The "Maintenance" clearly refers to the incomes of the wily state employees who administer the agency, inasmuch as many welfare recipients (sorry!) enjoy far less than a decently maintained income.

Have you bought a used car lately? Forget it. You won't find any. They are all "pre-owned" now.

I clearly remember the distinctive voice of Digby O'Dell,

your friendly undertaker, on *The Life of Riley* radio show. Alas, Digby is gone, along with all his fellow undertakers. Their places have been taken—but not necessarily filled—by Funeral Directors.

Come to think of it, no one dies anymore. We pass on, expire, cease breathing, go away, pass away, leave, or go to our own great rewards. Actually, dying is a much more dignified and simple act than passing on to your great reward. Not only is the reward debatable, it is, at best, uncertain. Dying is definite. Passing on is ambiguous and ill defined; it implies more, perhaps, than we want to know. Passing on to what? A more realistic great reward might be to donate our organs to the living.

Euphemism and obfuscation are methods by which we attempt to deal (rather ineffectively, it seems) with unpleasant problems. These problems won't go away just because we play word games.

The American medical community is getting knee-deep in acronyms, which can be defined as government-sponsored obfuscation. We now have State Health Planning and Development Agencies (SHPDAs), Statewide Health Coordinating Councils (SHCCs) and Health System Agencies (HSAs) that have been developed by the National Health Planning and Resources Development Act (NHPRDA). Health Maintenance Organizations (HMOs) are federally funded prepaid group practices. Local Health Care Providers (LHCPs) require a Certificate of Need (CON) in order to be paid by the Health Care Financing Administration (HCFA). Let me reiterate. Under NHPRDA, SHPDHs, SHCCs and HSAs, with HMOs, require a CON for LHCPs under the HCFA. Right? Got it? Of course, it's ridiculous. I think the whole program should be included in one giant agency called Department of Government Policy Options Operations Program (DOGPOOP), because dog poop is what it is.

Almost forty years ago, when the War Department became the Department of Defense, something terrible happened to us. We discovered the acceptability of doublethink and newspeak. I believe we have to resist further erosion of our language and our dignity. Garbagemen, maids, janitors, undertakers, doctors, lawyers and candlestick makers are all working for the general good of society. The unpleasant tasks we must perform will not become more attractive because of semantic shenanigans. We are born, we deal the best we can with life, we die. Surely we are entitled to the respect of having our efforts recognized in understandable terms, rather than being depreciated by arbitrary and imprecise sugarcoating. Our own Tower of Babel is being built with a language that is designed to tell us nothing.

Remember collywobbles? I do, with nostalgic affection. If you ate something that disagreed with your intestinal tract, you got collywobbles. Unfortunately, no one gets collywobbles anymore. You get gastroenteritis. The new, fancier term is harder to spell and much less fun than the old. Also, gastroenteritis has a more serious, more ominous ring to it. You recover quite quickly from a humorous-sounding illness like collywobbles; ginger ale usually takes care of it. But gastroenteritis gives me the feeling that treatment is necessary and complicated.

The same holds true for grippe. Fifty years ago, you got the grippe and that pretty well described how you felt: feverish, achy, tired. In short, you were "in the grip" of an illness. Now you get something with the innocuous title of influenza, a beige-sounding illness that, as far as I'm concerned, feels like grippe but doesn't sound nearly as dramatic.

We seem to need to alter perfectly good words to suit a twentieth-century requirement which dictates that labels themselves must modify conditions so as to make them more acceptable. All through the New Testament, Jesus is referred to as King of the Jews. Today, he undoubtedly would be known as the radical leader of minority groups of the Jewish persuasion. Something gets lost here, and I'm not at all convinced that the new freight train of adjectives carries as much meaning as the more direct statement.

At our hospital, we no longer have Ward Clerks—those vital, dedicated people who keep things running and enable other professionals to give patient care. These hospital workers are now referred to as Unit Coordinators. As far as I know, they did not get raises commensurate with their impressive new titles.

Prep-school infirmaries and nursing homes in my community are now licensed as Health Care Facilities. I'm fighting the system. I persist in treating sick youngsters in the infirmary and admitting terminally aged people to the nursing home. I'm not fooled by this sugarcoated pill, and neither, I suspect, are the students with grippe or the old folks who realize that collywobbles are as faraway a memory as Baby Snooks and Arthur Godfrey.

Of course, part of the beauty of language—ours in particular—is its adaptiveness and changeability. I grew up with Victrolas, later changed to record players, then to hi-fi sets, and—finally—to stereo systems. As the technology changed, so did the names. But some old habits die hard: I confess that I still get the milk bottle, although it's long been a carton, from the icebox (the iceman hasn't been around for a while).

Have you seen a pididdle recently? In my high-school clan, being the first one on a date to see a car with one darkened headlight entitled the boy to a free kiss. I don't see pididdles anymore, although I find myself dreamily looking for them at night. Perhaps automobile headlights are more efficient now. If so, we are depriving our youth of a glorious opportunity to... Well, it seemed fun and risqué at the time.

Today's look is punk. The in-crowd toots coke. When relaxing, you veg out; when eating candy, you carb out. Even though the modern generation may seem spaced-out, it appears able to coin meaty and descriptive expressions. We could take a linguistic cue from the young.

As grown-ups, we are at risk of cleansing our language to the point where it tells us nothing. War becomes defense, financial debt becomes a negative investment impact, curing the sick becomes a health maintenance mode. We tend to dump good words that tell us something and are, at the same time, exciting to read and pleasing to the ear.

How did we come to this sorry state of affairs? We have to go back to A.D. 1066 when the Battle of Hastings pitted a smaller and better-equipped Norman army against the Saxon defenders.

In a famous all-day battle, manners and language were forever altered. The etiquette of a French Norman court attained preference over the customs and speech of earthy Anglo-Saxons who, unfortunately, lost the historic struggle. As a result, words like "fornication," "defecation," "urination" and "regurgitation"—all suitable, polite French words—took the place of one-syllable Saxon terms with which we are all familiar because of their presence on john—excuse me, bathroom—walls. The Latin influence became inescapable in medical words like "feces" and "flatulence." Greek roots supplanted the insolent northern European terms: for example, diarrhea, leukorrhea, rhinorrhea and a formidable collection of other beige expressions that are favored by doctors but have to be looked up in dictionaries by motivated laymen.

Not only are Latin and Greek words more polite, they add to the mystery of medicine by sounding erudite and proper. In the final analysis, body functions are pretty well understood by everyone. I wonder if it really helps the patient to know she has leukorrhea (a vaginal discharge) or rhinorrhea (a snotty nose). Yet doctors are more comfortable putting fancy names on things. Somehow, it seems more genteel to call a case of clap by its Latinized name: gonoccal urethritis.

As a profession, doctors are scybalous. Now, before you stop reading right here, go to your dictionary (Webster's unabridged will do) and search for the word "scybalous." It is a beautiful term because it is so seemly, so decorous—a perfect example of what I am driving at. Were I to claim that most doctors are chock-full of the Saxon equivalent of scybala, I would be drummed out of the profession. The air would mysteriously leave the tires of my station wagon as it nestled unobtrusively in the hospital parking lot. Editors would not publish my columns. There would be a great hue and cry. Anything I wrote would automatically be removed from the newsstands. Alas, the reading public has become the true victim of the Battle of Hastings.

Doctors are scybalous for a variety of reasons, a prime one being that we happily cover up issues and take delight in obfuscation. We don't talk English; we talk fancy. We prefer words and explanations that sound refined but may not communicate our meaning.

I'll never forget hearing the best professor of endocrinology I ever knew tell a patient, a Puerto Rican who barely understood basic English, that the unfortunate immigrant had "hypoadren-ocorticism" for which treatment would require "evaluation of diurnal cortisol secretion." The doctor might just as well have been talking Greek; in fact, he was. Like the rest of us, the illustrious professor was hiding behind language; he felt safe there. The patient, in his ignorance, was miserable. How much more effective would have been an approach in which the physician explained the problem in terms intelligible to a medically unsophisticated person.

As a favor to your doctor, please don't ever leave his office until you have been given a simple and understandable explanation of what may be wrong with you. If enough patients continue to ask questions, someday we all may be able to talk to one another without having to deal with an excretory collection of scybala.

CHAPTER 11

THE
THIRD
AGE

THE THIRD AGE

❖

Some writers suffer the tortures of the damned in attempting to find synonyms for the term "old age." It sounds so hopeless and final that many people prefer euphemisms, such as "the golden age." The elderly may be referred to as "senior citizens," but aging is aging; the old get older.

The French, in their wonderfully Gallic way, seem to have less trouble with old age, at least in print. They classify life into three categories: the First Age is childhood, the Second Age is adulthood, and the Third Age is, well, old age. There may not be much promise as we reach the growing ranks of the elderly, but there is hope. So, the title of this chapter on aging is "The Third Age," because it seems to be a gentle term. Also, it suggests a flow of time, a natural progression from the First and Second ages. I like the term, and I thank the French for having invented it.

DEAR SON

❖

DEAR SON,

This nursing home isn't bad, as nursing homes go. On my 76th birthday last week, they gave me a cupcake with six candles. I got my first issue of *The Saturday Evening Post*, which you gave me. Judging from my copy, I must say it certainly isn't the same as it was in the 1940s, with wonderful stories like Alexander Botts and his tractor. Hasn't Norman Rockwell died yet? Whatever happened to *National Review*?

Why do I have to be in a place with so many old people? I don't feel old. I would much prefer to see more youngsters, like my grandchildren or the candy stripers in the hospital. The other residents seem to be preoccupied with three subjects: the past, how to get home, and their bowel habits. Do you think it was fair to put me here?

After lunch on Wednesday, I wrapped my dentures in the paper napkin on my tray. Before I could say "Teddy Roosevelt," a woman whisked away the remains of my meal, dentures and all. I hollered a lot, until they put a hold on the compactor and got my choppers. The whole experience was dehumanizing. I like that word. Dehumanizing. I read it in the large-type *Reader's Digest* I swiped from Mr. Abernathy. His glasses make his eyes seem so big he looks like a giant praying mantis from a science-fiction moving picture.

To be frank, I am not happy here. I know that the oil bills for heating my big house last winter were quite large, and I am truly sorry I almost set myself on fire with delinquent sparks from my pipe.

I think I should tell you we are required to arise and eat breakfast at 7 A.M. If the good Lord had meant for us to wake up at such a disgraceful hour, wouldn't He have made the sun come up earlier? I am not permitted to turn on the TV after 10 P.M. Therefore, I miss all the good old movies I'd love to watch. I spent most of my life working for money. Is this how my money should work for me?

I think I am truly the only healthy person in this place. I want a stiff drink. I object to being told when to bathe. Since I can no longer work in the yard every day, what difference does bathing make?

Oh, I guess it's okay here. Bridge. Sermons by that genteel minister from the local church. Bible-study classes. Flower arranging. Lectures on growing houseplants. But, as you can see, it's not like living by yourself. I miss your mother.

When the nursing-wing residents are lined up in their wheelchairs every morning to watch the talk shows on TV, they fall asleep. No one really watches TV. The picture and sound track simply provide a background for the desperately quiet act of growing old. Whoever termed old age as the "golden years" was nuts.

My joints ache. I have no appetite for bland food that has been cooked to death. I cannot control my body. I am perpetually embarrassed by those around me. I feel alone. I am slipping away and I want someone to care. Please help me.

Can you visit on Sunday? Bring Tollhouse cookies and Scotch. I have nothing to look forward to anymore.

Love,
DAD

IF YOU CAN'T RUN, WALK

I'm angry at my ten-speed bicycle; it prevents me from climbing hills as readily as I could a year ago. I'm ticked off at publishers in general; they are printing books, newspapers and magazines with such infuriatingly tiny type that I now must use the reading glasses I once reserved only for scanning the small print on insurance forms. I'm peeved at my hedge clippers; last month, while pruning a bush, I threw my back out and walked around for two days as though I were ... as though I were ... fifty years old. I get fed up at clothing manufacturers who mark waistbands 34 when they know they are 30; I always wore a 30 and I don't think they're fair to change sizes without warning me. I'm provoked at the makers of tennis courts who, after a perfectly benign acquiescence to the rules of the USLTA, suddenly decided to make courts wider and longer. As a result, I tire after three sets, when I used to be able to go five.

While a part of me acknowledges that I am growing older—after all, everyone does—I am surprised to see little skin crin-

kles at the corners of my shifty eyes. I don't see why I can't
play the great American game: Blame Your Woes on Others. I
don't feel old—usually; therefore, my diminishing physical re-
serve must be the fault of external factors: the military-industrial
complex, acid rain, Japanese cars, junk food, pipe smoking,
sunshine and the plethora of victimizers who waylay us oldies,
like the bears in A. A. Milne who "wait at the corners all ready
to eat the sillies who tread on the lines of the street. . . ."

The aging process appears to be inexorable. And one of the
responsibilities doctors have is to help make the process more
bearable. I believe in the necessity of remaining as active as
possible, while keeping in mind the natural restrictions of age.
If you can't run, walk. If you can't swim, wallow. If you can no
longer hit those booming forehand winners, be content with the
angled slice that will severely distress your younger opponent.
Use a golf cart if you have to, but—by heaven—continue to
play the game.

The question is not whether you are growing old. Rather,
it's whether you can make age work for you. Adapt. Slow down.
Make the other guy try harder. Enjoy physical activity to the
extent you can.

The same principle holds true for mental potency. Stay active. The problem is that the powers of memory tend to wane
with age. Now, with respect to memory loss . . . hmmm . . . I forget what I wanted to say.

PLAYING "THE GIN GAME"

❖

The Gin Game, a Pulitzer prize-winning drama by D. L. Coburn, starred Hume Cronyn and Jessica Tandy when it ran on Broadway and recently aired on public television. The play is devastating in its surgical dissection of an elderly unmarried couple in a nursing home. The humor of the first act relentlessly progresses into a tragic evisceration in which the characters claw and flail at each other to an exhausting denouement of futile loneliness and isolation.

The play is not a paean to old age. Nursing-home occupants are described as "rows of wrinkled pumpkinheads" inhabiting a "warehouse for the emotionally and intellectually dead." The elderly are portrayed as vicious and enraged people whom age and experience only embittered. Rather than soothing our deepest demons of hate and loathing, the aging process is shown to intensify our desolation, as independence and self-esteem—Coburn's antidotes for anger and frustration—wither. "First I made the mistake of getting sick," the protagonist explains, "then I made the mistake of getting well."

This is a far cry from what we romanticize old age to be: a dignified running down; silver-haired grandmothers bouncing fat babies on their knees, bespectacled elderly widowers still vital and useful after retirement.

My experience with older people has convinced me that the unhappy couple in *The Gin Game* is typical of only a small segment of the elderly. The ones I know do not regard their present lives as wastelands. They have managed to retain perspective and the capacity to adapt. Of course, senility is another issue. A profound loss of mental capability is a dreadful burden, one that we as a society have thus far failed to relieve.

For the average aging person, three realities seem paramount. Related in some ways, these factors are nonetheless independent of one another.

First, older people feel a loss of control. During our adulthood, most of us try in one way or another to control ourselves and our environment. We organize households, earn livelihoods, raise children. We create. We interact with others, organize our lives and get about the business of living. We shop, plan and supervise. We go to the movies or for an automobile drive when we feel like doing so. We have mastered our bodily functions and, in general, we can take care of ourselves.

As we age, however, we sense an erosion of our control. We have less to say about our lives; fewer people listen to us. We become physically weaker and depend more on others. We have bladder and bowel problems. We can't see as well, think as clearly or run our lives as efficiently as before. Our bodies begin to fail us, although we may still feel "young."

As we progressively lose control, the control is assumed by others and our perception of helplessness grows. If we live long enough, we may eventually have to be taken care of in nursing homes, where we abdicate our most basic levels of control: eating, sleeping, eliminating. Not a cheering prospect.

Second, the elderly may feel isolated. Their friends have died; their children and grandchildren may have moved away or emotionally distanced themselves. The world moves too fast, things are difficult to learn all over again, and life becomes paralyzingly complicated. For a variety of reasons—some of them valid—society encourages this isolation. Families put ailing relatives into nursing homes. Aunt Rose may be getting the nutritional meals she was unable to prepare for herself, but she is being deprived of a crucial resource she and all other people need: contact with the larger world. Nursing homes may be great places, but there are no young people residing in them.

In these instances, the aged are denied the stimulating variations of younger adults and children. There is nothing lonelier for an older person than other lonely older people. I would like to see more widespread adoption of a system that has proved successful in many parts of the country: frequent visits by grade-school children to old-age homes. It's a valuable experience for the youngsters and really makes the older people's eyes light up.

The third fundamental is fear. The elderly fear many things: death, dying, pain, illness, dependency and growing older. They also fear loss of control and isolation. I think that we younger folks—especially doctors—have to take more account of this fear.

It's real, it's palpable and it's part of aging. For some physicians, treating the elderly is an intolerable task. Doctors-in-training will often refer to aged patients (with a plethora of medical problems) as "crocks" or "gomers" (for "Get Out of My Emergency Room!"). Heroic treatment is sometimes viewed as prolonging the inevitable. On the other hand, advanced life support may be slavishly exercised for training purposes in teaching hospitals, to the detriment of the patient.

We must learn to help the elderly with their fears, using as much determination as we devote to their ailing hearts. I'd like to see every older person who arrives in an emergency room or doctor's office wear a T-shirt that proclaims; "Don't be too harsh, my dear; your time will come soon enough!"

Aging may, on occasion, seem to bring with it the desperation portrayed in *The Gin Game*, but it doesn't have to be that way. The success with which the elderly cope with aging may reflect the ways in which they can learn to adapt to a variety of issues. For our part, we younger people and physicians need to empathize with elderly people's perceptions, sympathize with their needs and provide the courtesy of treating them as we ourselves will want to be treated in the future.

THE ELUSIVE FOUNTAIN OF YOUTH

❖

The civilized world for several years has been intrigued with the possibility of tricking Mother Nature. However, as we learned from the margarine advertisements on television, it's not nice to fool her. The old girl herself usually has the last laugh. Case in point: longevity.

In the late 1960s, certain mountain people—notably, residents of the remote Ecuadorian village of Vilcambaba, in the Andes, and two isolated villages in the Soviet Caucasus—were discovered to have achieved a seemingly remarkable old age. An extremely high number of villagers claimed to be over sixty years of age; a few had reached astounding ages exceeding one hundred.

Researchers were baffled about the factors permitting such longevity. Was it mountain air? Diet? Goat's milk? Strenuous exercise? Tension-free life-style? Genes? Intricate analyses showed no identifiable fountain of youth. The waters of scientific investigation were further muddied when centenarians were found to enjoy substantial quantities of alcohol, dairy-product diets and strong, evil-smelling tobacco. The old people walked a great deal—an understandable necessity in areas where transportation was limited—but appeared, in most respects, to have living patterns typical of agricultural communities. After years of study and head scratching, eminent doctors from the United States and the Soviet Union concluded that a combination of genetic inheritance and frugal, vigorous, nontechnological life-style was the probable common denominator for longevity. The investigators' results were duly reported in books and reputable journals.

According to *Time*, a tiny craze in the ceramic of research appeared in the mid-1970s. Dr. Alexander Leaf, an American physician, had interviewed in 1970 a Vilcambaba oldster who gave his age as 121. When reinterviewed by Dr. Leaf in 1974, the centenarian claimed an age of 132.

With that flash of insight that occasionally illuminates medical discovery, Dr. Leaf performed some rapid calculations and concluded that either the Andean mountain air was getting to him or he had been conned. Returning to the proverbial drawing board—in this case, baptismal records—investigators discovered they had been royally bamboozled; the old people had lied about their ages. There wasn't a centenarian in the entire village. The oldest resident was a mere ninety-six. The old folks had lied in hopes of attracting tourist dollars to their out-of-the-way village. Apparently, Russian scientists discovered the same embarrassing truth when they reinvestigated their own old-age groups in the Caucasus.

Aside from the obvious conclusion that even reputable scientists make mistakes, what should we have learned from these events? Two thoughts come to mind.

First, we had better be wary of accepting statements at face value. We must be more discriminating in what we embrace as Truth. The pontifical pronouncements of so-called learned men have, historically, not always been the last—or even the correct—word. One of the most precious prerogatives of free men is the right to question. And if there was ever a need to exercise that right, it is right now—in our media-saturated, communications-worshipping, authority-figured twentieth-century society.

The second thought on the subject of longevity is obviously better suited to biology. Man's life-span seems to be narrowly finite. Barring accidents, disease and (the very real) future possibility of genetic engineering, each of us would probably tend to wear out at about the same age, give or take a decade. Exercise, proper diet, spiritual nourishment and avoidance of a deleterious environment are all factors that can improve the quality of life but not necessarily its length. The aging process itself appears to be securely and genetically controlled. In other words, the phenomenon called "dying of old age" affects all

persons at about the same time in life. The upward manipulation
of that age is presently beyond the scope of our knowledge. Alas,
the El Dorado of youthfulness is not to be found in the Andes
or the Caucasus. The antidote for aging will more likely issue
from a shiny, sparkling laboratory than from a shiny, sparkling
fountain.

Until the day we are blessed—or cursed—with a pill to pep
up our tired DNA, we might better spend our time figuring out
how we can cram more into our allotted span. And, by all means,
thoroughly check the birth certificates of centenarians.

PRISM OF AUTUMN: THREE REFLECTIONS

❖

There's Good News and Bad News:
Have you ever wondered why time
seems to pass so slowly when we are
young and flash by so quickly as we
age? The answer may be an arithmetic
ratio: the relation of unit time to total
life-span. For example, to a child of
six, a year is one-sixth of his life; to
a person of sixty, a year is one-sixtieth.
Therefore, a year appears to pass much
more rapidly for an oldster than it does
for a youngster. I have termed this
insight Williams' Theorem, in honor of Carl Williams, a math-
ematics teacher at Salisbury School, who first brought the phenomenon to my attention.

The speed with which time passes is, of course, only an
incidental observation. There are more important considerations. As we age, our perspectives change, our minds and bodies
mature—and then decline. It has been said that a man of forty
has half the physical capability of a youth of twenty; by age
sixty, he has half the capability he had at forty. This fact seldom
causes wild rejoicing among older folks. But the message is
clear: our physical skills begin to fade in our twenties and

continue to follow a progressively downhill slope as long as we live.

Somatic abilities aside, I get the feeling that what we all dread most is the inevitable mental decline. Issues of judgment, memory and emotional control—the basic requirements for living in society—seem so obscenely taken for granted by young adults. The falloff of mental acuity presents not only practical problems but, often, sheer panic to the elderly. A failing brain, in conjunction with an unpredictable body, is an enormous burden for patients and families to bear. Although most people can be kept alive—in institutions—long after they have ceased to be normally functioning human beings, I doubt that most of us relish such an ignominious conclusion to our lives.

In the *New England Journal of Medicine*, Dr. Sidney Katz and his colleagues have reawakened an interest in defining the length of *useful* existence for aging people. Like most conclusions, their findings contain both bad news and good.

To begin with, they point out that standard actuarial tables, which use death as an end point, are misleading. Instead, the authors prefer a concept of Active Life Expectancy: the length of time an individual can expect to maintain reasonable independence. Independence is defined in terms of whether a person can feed, bathe, and dress himself and is minimally mobile in transferring himself from bed to chair.

Active Life Expectancy is, predictably, less than the traditional and simpler Life Expectancy. Yet it tells a great deal more, and will, the authors hope, enable health agencies to determine more realistically what the precise needs of a progressively aging population are.

First, the bad news: Each person appears to have a biological life of about eighty-five years. Yes, this is an average and there are exceptions to the figure. But, by and large, the human machine wears out after eighty-five to ninety years. Until our genes can be spliced, most of us have to accept that limit and make the best of it.

Now, the good news: Medical science is making tremendous

progress in controlling the chronic diseases that cause people to wear out, or become functionally dependent before they have reached their biological limit. More and more physicians are directing their attention to improving the quality of older people's lives, rather than simply emphasizing prevention of death. Doctors are looking more closely at ways to help oldsters remain useful and productive, if possible—or, at least, independent. Natural death may not be the enemy; chronic and enervating dependency is the opponent to be conquered. Life may be slipping—or rushing—by, but we can take heart. There is hope that the disabling diseases of brain and body can be overcome. The end result may well be an elderly person who is able to remain functionally independent until the moment when his genetic clock fails.

Living Longer Is Not Always Living Well: My father was reminiscing the other day about the tremendous change in the past sixty years with respect to the concept of what constitutes Good Health. In bygone times, men were "portly." A paunchy stomach was considered socially necessary. My great-uncle Charles used to fall asleep regularly after his traditional Sunday midday cocktail and roast beef dinner. Plethoric, with his face the color of a ripe plum, he monopolized the living-room easy chair. As he snoozed, the lighted cigar in his mouth dribbled flakes of gray ash upon his ample, waistcoated abdomen. He died, my father remembered, in his late sixties, presumably of a heart attack. Precise diagnosis was unfashionable in those days. My grandmother, a kind and abstemious soul, was said to have died of acute indigestion after having eaten too much French toast. As a result, this breakfast delicacy was forbidden in my father's house during his childhood.

Years ago, women were considered attractive if they were "stout." However, no self-respecting lady would be caught dead in public unless she had been furled into her corset. I am not referring to the anemic latex supports sported by today's "full-figured" matrons. I am talking about those glorious antique corsets of muslin, whalebone and incredibly complex arrangement of laces, which, when finally in place, made their wearers look like stiff hourglasses that could not breathe.

A man was judged by his peers in terms of how much he liked to eat and drink. In middle age, you disdained athletic endeavor—except, perhaps, to walk to the streetcar on the way to work. The purpose of life was to enjoy what you could. Meals rich in cholesterol—roast beef, sauces, pies, pastry, butter, eggs, heavy cream—were the norm. Cancer was a curiosity. Nursing homes were practically nonexistent. Dietary prohibitions were minimal.

This picture of the early twentieth-century citizen would be anathema to today's compulsively health-conscious consumer. Millions of sweating, grim, tight-lipped runners clog our byways in order to experience the daily pain considered necessary in the latest attempt to prolong life—the new Fountain of Youth.

We are afraid to eat too much. We execrate eating the Wrong Thing, whatever that may be at a given moment. Exercise has become as important to us as churchgoing was to our grand-parents—and it is probably not much more effective in maintaining good health. We experience hideous dreams about energy crises, nuclear Armageddon and the evils of cold breakfast cereal. We analyze everything; boy, do we analyze. Who am I? What is happiness? What can I do to prevent boredom? Learn the answers in the latest book written by a self-proclaimed expert.

Somewhere along the line, we seem to have lost the ability to enjoy life, the tremendous variety of experiences available to us. Nursing homes have long waiting lists and cannot accommodate a burgeoning number of elderly, temperate, frugal patients whose hearts and kidneys are functioning fine, thank you, but whose brains have been so mildewed by senility that these long-lived dear people don't even know they exist on the planet earth.

I don't mean to sound cruel, nor do I wish to depreciate the marvelous medical advances that have saved so many of our young, particularly children. But we are missing something; that something may be Fun. Maybe even—God forbid—Meaning.

One fact is abundantly clear. Our social resources have yet to catch up to our scientific achievements. We appear to be more concerned with questions of pure longevity than with the more central issue: How to cram more style into our lives.

Lewis Thomas has written that if we could mimic the famous One-Horse Shay and arrange for everything to fall apart at once— preferably on our one-hundredth birthdays—our lives would become immeasurably simpler. But that is not to be, I am afraid. We will, embarrassingly, continue to wear out in little bits and pieces.

Perhaps we need to accept that fact. Living a long time may not be synonomous with enjoying what time we have. Of course, a few of us seem to choose to shorten our lives unnecessarily by being foolishly extreme and self-destructive. However, I believe we can honestly ask the basic question: What purpose do we serve by eschewing even a moderate life-style if we are eventually relegated to a nursing home because we have aged too greatly to be able to take care of ourselves? Would we not be infinitely better off to be able to say at the end: "Thank you; I have had a lovely time." Now that's style.

Nantucket in October: I have tended to regard Nantucket, Massachusetts, as a summer vacation spot. The island in July is a brown-legged girl with skirts held high, smelling of roses and privet. She is youth and sunshine as she wriggles her toes in the hot sand of a rutted, dusty back road. She revels in the pleasure of early-morning sea mist that burns off during long and languid summer afternoons. She is optimism, vitality, sparkling exuberance; her laugh is the sweet song of tiny birds. She wears sea grapes in her hair.

This past October my wife and I journeyed to the island to discover the "other" Nantucket. The gray-shingled beach houses were boarded up; the moors were a collage of russet, red and purple. A cold drizzle from the sea blew in over deserted cobble-stone streets. The scent of flowers had given way to the smells of wet leaves and woodsmoke. My raucous sunshine girl had changed into a serene woman. More properly, she had grown and developed. In the course of a few weeks, this tiny windswept retreat had passed from gregarious adolescence to sedate middle age. This caused me to reflect on the difficult task we humans have in accepting the inevitability of change and aging.

We are a society obsessed with youthfulness. Healthy adults spend fortunes on medical procedures that are designed to make us appear younger. We resort to creams, lotions, moisturizers, mudpacks, face-lifts, chin-tucks and a variety of cosmetics to cover the obvious signs of age. We exercise to exhaustion in vain attempts to unclog plugged pipes. We take hormones, wear pastel clothes, follow the sun, gobble vitamins . . . and then complain that our bodies can't do what they could thirty years ago. We forget that we can't, in fact, reverse the aging process— even with shots, ointments and gels. The biological clock is built in, right there, ticking away despite all our tricks and denials.

We could approach the inevitability of growing older with an eye cocked to an unyielding nature that teaches us to let go of the seasons and enjoy the changes that are programmed into every living cell. After all, to the experienced observer, the flashy vigor of summer is no more radiant than the visual cacophony of fall. But this view seems too rhetorical. What middle-aged adult could reasonably be satisfied with what my father calls "the lengthening shadows"? The fact is, we want to remain young. More precisely, we wish to radiate *the image* of being young.

I am told that in Japan, commuters will smile when they miss a subway train. They are disappointed, but not frustrated, because they feel that events are unfolding in proper order. The subway was scheduled to leave at a certain moment, and the delayed commuter obtains satisfaction from realizing that the natural course of events is proceeding on a predictable and appropriate schedule. It's very Zen, but we Westerners have a long way to go before we adopt such profound reverence for the order of things.

What we seem to hanker for in our fast-food culture is an elusive quality called Class. Class isn't something you obtain by eating in the right restaurant, wearing the right clothes or cultivating the right friends. You can't develop it by reading the right books, although certain authors make a substantial living by convincing you that you can.

Class is a way of looking at life that sometimes comes to people as they age. Children don't have Class, but many adults do, simply because of experience and, perhaps, the realization that the aging process can't be denied, bargained against or cheated.

We all covet Class, but we're reluctant to commit ourselves to certain inevitabilities in order to get it. Growing old gracefully is classy. No one can tell you how to do it. But we all know people who do. Taking a subway in Tokyo and missing your connection—then smiling—may help. If you can't manage a trip to the Orient next year, how about Nantucket in October?

CHAPTER 12

AND NOBODY GETS OUT ALIVE

ICEBERG QUESTIONS

❖

Colorado Governor Richard Lamm created quite a stir in 1984 when he took the position that government can no longer afford to subsidize medical costs for the elderly who are terminally ill. Among other things, the governor observed that old people are like "leaves falling and forming humus for the other plants to grow." They should not have their lives "artificially extended," he said. "They have a duty to die and get out of the way" of "the other society, our kids."

Now, I can appreciate Lamm's concern about the cost of health care. We are all aware of dire predictions that the Medicare program will be insolvent by the 1990s. We realize that there are financial limits beyond which government cannot afford to trespass. Anybody who can read knows that federal and state medical funding is already in trouble, and that problems are multiplying at an unacceptable rate.

Yet—and this is a big "yet"—do we really want to embrace a put-'em-out-on-the-iceberg philosophy? At the rate at which we are living longer, this country will experience, within a few years, a two- or threefold increase in the number of people aged sixty and older. Like youngsters, the aged tend to get sick more often. They need surgery—often major surgery, like coronary bypass or organ transplants. So medical care for the senescent costs more. A quiet and relatively painless death, unlike spring sunshine, doesn't come when it's most needed.

However, I harbor a multitude of objections to allowing death to become a political issue. For one thing, I sure as heck don't want a bureaucrat with a computer telling me or a member of my family when to die. Despite the allure of stainless-steel machines, they are not the solution to the moral-ethical questions

that rattle the windows of our society. Somewhere, we have got
to keep the decision making on a personal level.

In today's culture, even that may not be enough. Patients
with no possible hope of living a meaningful existence are scan-
dalously being kept alive by well-meaning doctors and families
who wrongly assign death the role of adversary. Our problem is
simple: Medical science has the technology and wherewithal to
extend life almost indefinitely. Of course, the cost in money and
dehumanization is paralyzing. The answers are complex; we still
don't know them all, and in many cases, we cannot even grasp
the enormity of the issues. One fact seems clear: The patient's
wishes are often ignored. Through some gigantic shell-and-pea
game, his preferences get lost along the way.

I suspect that most hospitals in this republic contain at least
one elderly valetudinarian who is, in the current jargon, the
recipient of a total life-support system. The heart is beating, the
lungs are inflating, the kidneys are excreting, the body is feeding
... all through the wondrous courtesy of sparking electrodes,
huffing respirators, plastic gizmos, tubes and more tubes. Aunt
Ella is, by the grace of God and the medical profession, alive;
but she is in a deep coma and could no more recognize the
Sunday newspaper than she could breakdance.

Where do we go from here? Aunt Ella is old enough to carbon
date, lived in seclusion for the last ten years of her life (since
Uncle Leonard "passed" after his second hernia operation) and
long ago depleted the annuity from her War Bonds. She has
been machine-dependent for six months, and no one knows how
to resolve the issue. The doctor can't pull the plug; he'd be in
court before the funeral was over. The guilt-ridden family stands
pat; what layman feels comfortable about making a death decision? The hospital welcomes the income from a "utilized" bed.

You may have guessed by now that I don't have any answers
either, except to suggest that Aunt Ella—and the countless
others like her—has, like everyone else, always needed at least
a little independence. Perhaps the critical decisions about her
future should have been made within the first few days of her
hospitalization. And with her consent and full approval; ideally,

while she had enough mental acuity to make a rational decision—before she became ill, in fact. The longer these things are put off, the harder they may become to deal with.

Flexibility. Consultation with family and clergy. Open communication. No artificial life support without hope of recovery. Above all, acquiescence to the patient's wishes. Are these the answers? Does anyone know? But at least we are talking and thinking about the problem. It's your decision—your decision it's got to be. People are *not* just humus; each human "leaf" is important and unique.

WHEN THE CHIPS FALL

Not long ago, I made a house call on an octogenarian gentlewoman. (Yes, Virginia, doctors do still make house calls.) She was suffering from a particularly unpleasant condition called acute pulmonary edema, in which inefficient heart action causes excessive fluid accumulation within the lungs. This highly intelligent lady was experiencing severe respiratory difficulty, and as I prepared to give her an injection, she sighed: "At my age, I have resigned myself to letting the chips fall as they may, but I don't want them to fall *this* way!"

After a couple of days in the hospital, she was comfortable enough to return home to her normal routine. However, her statement has been skittering around in my brain and has caused me to reflect on questions of how and when people die.

To be candid, we all want a painless death that comes when we are prepared and that involves a minimum of discomfort and trouble for others. Ideally, we hope to die at a relatively old age, preferably in our sleep. A satisfactory alternative for some of us would be to succumb to a heart attack, as my grandfather did, quietly, on the ninth hole, under a tree, waiting for a rain shower to pass. Often people die quite quickly in a state of coma following cardiac arrest, massive strokes or serious accidents. Those intellectually honest patients who sign Living Wills do so with the conviction that they will not relish being burdens to their families, friends and communities if, in fact, there is no chance of returning to a useful life. Most human beings abhor the thought of ending up as a "vegetable," hooked to shiny machines that automatically carry on life support for a victim who will never again appreciate the smells of a sunny July morning or the taste of an English muffin slathered with strawberry jam. No one can fault the wishes of an old person who has lived a long and productive life, cannot conceive of total dependency and simply desires to be left alone to die in peace.

Yet there is a hitch in this system; the chips don't always fall as we would like them to. Death comes in unexpected ways, sometimes with startling clarity, usually with surprise, almost always with pain. We cannot call the shots. We are helpless and vulnerable. The dying patient may be "ready" for the end—but not this kind of end. Although each of us desperately hopes to avoid suffering, pain and dependency, doctors often see patients' beliefs changing when they realize they may be in a terminal state. Our reactions are as unique as our fingerprints, and just about as mystifying.

Families, doctors and hospitals must be made aware of the patient's wishes. At the same time, we should be ready to individualize, depending on circumstances. Above all, we must attempt to relieve the patient's pain, both physical and emotional. The total person has to be considered. That is the heart of medical practice and must never be relinquished, either to machines or to the power of the state. Death is never easy, but much of the suffering and discomfort associated with it can be ameliorated. The wonders of modern hospitals are not enough. Clergy, the love of family, and the many resources available to the patient must be brought into play and coordinated so that the sick person's needs and wishes are constantly being identified and monitored. Although the chips may have to fall, they don't have to drop with a clatter.

THE LAST JOURNEY

❖

Of all the enemies doctors are taught to dread—cancer, heart disease, incapacitation, illness—none equals death. For us, the death of our patients is our ultimate failure, the proof of our vulnerability, the adversary we learn to fear and abhor most. On our rounds as young white-coated saviors, during our exhausting all-night vigils with the sick, as interns and residents—gleaming with optimism, bursting with arrogance and overconfidence—we are programmed to despise death. To the new practitioner, death is a painful eventuality to be cheated, put off, prevented at any cost.

Is it possible we may have been wrong?

The experienced physician learns, with time, that death need not be a sinister evil to be conquered hand-to-hand in the sickroom—a bareknuckled contest at the bedside or a complicated war using all the weapons of twentieth-century medicine. Death may, in certain instances, be preferable to a goalless, painful, inhumane, stagnant existence. Rather than being the enemy, death may be a friend, a single, brilliant facet of life's jewel.

Years ago, I was privileged to have under my care a remarkable man who was dying of terminal and incurable cancer. He told me: "You know, Doc, it's not the dying that bothers me; it's the getting there that's hard." Judging from the current interest in Living Wills, many people seem to agree that death is not to be feared once reasonable (albeit unsuccessful) medical efforts to sustain life have been exhausted. Social issues aside, perhaps the greatest service a doctor can perform is to minimize

pain and relieve suffering in the terminally ill in order to prepare
the dying patient to pass into that silent realm we, the living,
so often fear.

I say that because in the past few years we have come to
understand more about the act of dying. It may not be as terrible
a defeat as we have been led to believe.

To begin with, death may not be particularly frightening and
uncomfortable. Patients who have "died"—from cardiac arrest,
for example—and been resuscitated tell us that they experienced, at the end, a suffusive feeling of tremendous peace; some
report seeing a golden light at the end of a tunnel. They describe
overwhelmingly pleasurable sensations of well-being, self-
knowledge, oneness and relaxation. They often detail an
eerie—but, to them, perfectly normal—awareness of talking to
long-dead relatives and loved ones. Many resuscitated patients
are disappointed at having been "brought back" to life.

Apparently our brains are able to prepare us for the ultimate.
Some experts in the field of thanatology—the study of death—
believe that during a person's last moments, brain tissue secretes
several natural opiates—endorphins—to facilitate the final pas-
sage from life to death. These compounds affect us in marvelous
ways to block pain, fear and guilt, so the dying patient may
accept death without the horrendous concomitants we, the living,
project onto the act.

The endorphins are truly remarkable chemicals. I have been
told by war veterans that when they were struck with shrapnel
or bullets, the only sensations they felt were surprise and a
feeling of numbness in the damaged area. Endorphins. Massive
injury, with blood loss and shock, rarely produces excruciating
pain.

Now researchers have discovered that the euphoria, or "high,"
experienced by long-distance runners may be the result of endorphins released during prolonged physical exertion. What a
miracle! At times of greatest stress, the body has been endowed
with a method to blunt pain.

No one in his right mind would suggest that doctors—or
anybody else, for that matter—should deliberately take mea-

sures to shorten the life of the patient. However, a natural ending need not be viewed as a terrifying event, fraught with agony and defeat. I am heartened by the knowledge that the living organism, with all its imperfections, has as standard equipment a means by which to alleviate the burden of passing from life, as we know it, to the next adventure.

MICHAEL'S DEATH

❖

Michael has died.

He was forty-six years old. From the time we were college classmates, he seemed superhuman: varsity football player, intellectual, Rhodes scholar, physician, poet, author, humanist, private-school and university trustee. An avid runner, he disdained alcohol and cigarettes, respected the gift of good health, and insisted on performing good works throughout his adult life.

I am told he died of cardiac arrest following surgery. He leaves a wife and several young children. His obscenely sudden and unexpected death underscores, for me, an important human fallacy that seems an integral part of Western civilization: we behave as though we control our lives.

I wonder if that fantasy helps explain our cultural abhorrence of death. We can somehow—although with difficulty—accept the loss of certain people: criminals and "evil" persons, the very elderly, the terminally ill, the hopelessly deformed and injured. However, when a person is picked, as is said, in the bloom of life, certain questions nuzzle to the forefront of consciousness. We are bewildered by a "divine plan," a "heartless God," the unpredictability of life. In fact, there may be no understandable reason for an untimely death, and perhaps we would do better to try to avoid seeking one. After all, philosophers have said that we know less about our universe than an ant knows about the British Museum. The concept of singularity, that pinpoint of time and space from which the cosmos was derived in a Big Bang, remains an idea only vaguely dreamed about by our greatest thinkers.

Orientals, as well as many primitive people, take the position that destiny is destiny. Wouldn't we be happier with our Western European, so-called civilized morality if we could stop asking questions that are painful and irrelevant? Acceptance of an inevitably chaotic and ambiguous existence may be the answer. Truth is simplicity.

When I mentioned Michael's death to a colleague whose opinions I value, he said we are all gnats on the windshield of life. This may seem flip; however, on reflection I see that this harsh metaphor expresses a certain vernacular profundity.

In the millions of years in which living species—including humanoids—have inhabited this planet, no creature appears to have been able unequivocally to determine the Sense of it all. Yes, I know that great religious prophets have made an effort to explain divine rationale. But saying "it is God's will" seems self-serving and childishly obvious. There is mystery here, more mysterious than we can grasp.

So, how does one deal with the premature death of a talented and multifaceted friend? The sadness may be lessened by realizing that there may be no understandable purpose, no recognizable pattern. Like many of life's inconsistent vicissitudes, it just happens. And it will continue to happen because we are powerless to comprehend, much less explain, the very nature of our existence. We don't even know the rules.

Yet our greatest strength may lie in our unique biological urge to question, pry and sort out. The irony could be that we have to explore the unfathomable in order to find meaning. We must continue to reach. Michael did. He understood.

CHAPTER 13

TWENTIETH-CENTURY MEDICINE AND THE HIGH-TECH FUTURE

❖

BIG MEDICINE DWARFS PEOPLE

❖

"You take the high road and I'll take the low road" is the first line of a well-known Scottish ditty. It might serve equally well as the opening sentence of a proclamation addressing medical care in the 1990s. This country, through its government agencies and industrial complex, seems increasingly more intent upon developing a two-tier system of health care. The reason for this abomination is profit; the name of the game is the Medical Industry.

In a 1985 issue of *Connecticut Medicine*, Professor Robert Massey, of the University of Connecticut School of Medicine, wrote: "Money has become the measure and profit the only legitimate goal in the world of the great corporate conglomerates; that medicine and the institutions of medicine should be following so rapidly and eagerly in that direction is unexpected and troubling." This orientation signals a startling shift in health-care policy. Doctors are being encouraged—at times, actually forced—to move from a humanistic-scientific approach to an industrial-economic posture.

In a March 1985 editorial in the *New England Journal of Medicine*, Dr. Steve Freedman of the University of Florida described "megacorporate health care" as the potential result of business, industry and government becoming active purchasers of medical care through Health Maintenance Organizations (HMOs) and Preferred Provider Organizations (PPOs). Some experts argue that medicine will ultimately be run by a huge combine of government, corporations and private insurance companies. Doctors, nurses, therapists, pharmacists—and most important, patients—will have little, if any, control over how, where and to what extent medical care will be delivered. High-level care will be available either to those who are very rich or who are covered by blanket cost-effective insurance. Other, less fortunate patients will not be covered and will be able to obtain only the most rudimentary level of medical attention. The traditional view of equal access for all citizens will metamorphose into a two-tier have-and-have-not system.

The effects of this brave new medical world are predictable: administrators will administrate; regulators will regulate; managers will manage. Doctors will become employees of huge profit-motivated companies; the healing arts will become secondary to rules prescribing appropriate "cost-effective" treatment. Medical education and research will dwindle because, as Dr. Freedman writes, they don't "preserve and enhance capital." The selling of medical skills will dominate over the improvement of those skills. Hospitals will relinquish humanitarian concerns in favor of discount-house, fast-food mentality. We will all be trapped in an enterprise whose sole concern is low-risk, big-return investment, rather than curing and caring for the sick and injured.

Dr. Freedman asks: "Can the practitioners resist the change? Yes, but only for a short time. The more important question is whether the large corporate and governmental purchasers who employ or provide support to the 'paying' consumers will wish to resist."

Does the average American really want pre-packaged medical care, faceless technology, Cabbage Patch doctors and institutional profitability? I think not. Medicine involves more than simple economic concerns and bureaucrats who ignore the complexities of health care. The values of trust, courtesy, caring and competence do not lend themselves to bottom-line ledger scratching.

I think it's fair to say that an astonishing majority of physicians disagrees with the concept of corporate megamedicine. The reasons are legion, but, in the final analysis, such a prospect means deterioration of patient care, and most doctors want to do a good job helping those they serve. Distant boardroom decisions can serve only to contaminate community needs and destroy the physician-patient relation, which, to many of us, is a vital part of the healing process. Nonetheless, young doctors (who have recently completed their training) are reported to be accustomed to institutionalized practice and "consequently will adapt readily to the corporate practice environment." The prospect is disquieting.

Medical practice today is unrecognizable from what it was forty, thirty, even twenty years ago. In many ways, the patient is better off; in some ways, not. Analysts are predicting more astounding alterations in the next decade or two. Surely, some of these modifications will be beneficial. But for those doctors and patients who bemoan the intrusion of government and industry into medical practice, the end is not in sight. As the old vaudeville saying has it, "You ain't seen nothin' yet."

IMPACTING ON UNCLE SAM

❖

At the risk of sounding self-serving, I'd like to inform the public that the Medicare system now classifies doctors into privileged and nonprivileged groups, haves and have-nots.

I'm not talking about the Cadillac/country-club specialist versus the Chevrolet/country practitioner. I'm referring to a more invidious distinction: those M.D.s who suck up to the government and those who don't.

It sounds peculiar, but it's true. Doctors who accept Medicare assignment are permitted to raise their fees for Medicare patients; physicians who don't accept a federal subsidy cannot. This through-the-looking-glass legislation is Uncle Sam's way of forcing every doctor to become dependent on Medicare payments.

Put another way, the system works like this: A doctor who "participates" in Medicare had previously agreed to accept for his services the very modest amount allowed by the government. This privileged physician is now permitted to increase his fees.

As far as I can determine, he can, if he wishes, triple or quadruple his charges; the sky's the limit, as it were. His cup runneth over.

On the other hand, the practitioner who does not participate in Medicare (and who may very well have voluntarily frozen his fees last year) is prohibited from increasing his charges to the levels enjoyed by his colleagues. If the doctor "willfully increases his charges," he is "subject to assessment of up to double the amount of the violation charges, civil money penalties (up to $2,000 per violation) and/or exclusion from the Medicare program for up to five years."

When looked at from a purely financial perspective, this have-and-have-not system doesn't make much sense. By permitting participating physicians to raise their fees, the bureaucrats are guaranteeing that Medicare reimbursement will rise across the board. More of our tax money will be spent, and the cost of Medicare will increase. But how can this be? It's a sticky situation.

The intelligent taxpayer may conclude that the purpose of this ploy is not financial, but psychological. It is a transparent trick to put all doctors under federal control—the old carrot-and-stick maneuver. Once you entice the sheep into the pen voluntarily, using food as bait, you've got them. The stick becomes unnecessary. You've made your roundup and you can do whatever you want to them.

I began by saying that I risked being considered self-serving. After all, few members of the public at large believe that doctors are underpaid. In fact, we are quite well paid. So the consumer may feel justified in asking: "What do I care about the doctors' tawdry fee dispute with the government?"

There is good reason to care, Mr. and Mrs. John Q. Patient, because—sooner or later—all these "cost-cutting" measures are going to trickle down and deeply affect you. You and your doctor are rapidly losing control of your health care, and at the rate things are going, it won't be long before most of that control is assumed by federal authorities.

Already, serious consideration is being given to a widespread plan for preadmission certification. This means that no patient over sixty-five will be electively admitted to a hospital without that admission being approved, in advance, by a bureaucrat. You will just have to put up with the pain of your kidney stone until 9 A.M., when the Medicare office opens and your doctor can begin the long paper-work battle to allow you to enter the hospital for relief. Sure, you might have pneumonia, but that won't necessarily entitle you to hospital treatment, even if you are eighty-three and live alone. Okay, so you might need hernia surgery—but you may have to wait several months until you can convince a government accountant with a green eyeshade that your hernia requires repair.

Esteemed patient, you and your doctor won't be making many decisions in the future. Your health and comfort will become the responsibility of some remote office worker who will reach judgments that are based on cost tables, profiles and print-outs. Medical care will become computerized and impersonal, a consumer product with all the individuality of a postage stamp. You will apply for hospitalization the way a candidate takes a civil-service examination. And tough luck if you don't make the grade. Your doctor won't be able to help you; he or she will be a paid, "privileged" participant in the system.

Is this what sick people really want?

In its tireless wisdom, the government—which means some darned fool—has created the Connecticut Peer Review Organization, Inc. This is known familiarly as CPRO, and if the name sounds like C3PO, the little robot in *Star Wars*, so be it. The difference is that C3PO makes more sense than CPRO.

Before you citizens settle down in amusement at what's happening in Connecticut these days, let me remind you that peer-review organizations are mandated for every state in the Union. They have different titles, but their purpose is the same: to decide which elderly patients can enter hospitals and which can't. These review organizations have the right to screen certain patients for hospital admission, and either to refuse Medicare reimbursement before the hospitalization or, in some cases, to refuse payment once the patients have been discharged. This is part of the federal cost-cutting compulsion.

The government fellas attempted to legitimize CPRO by putting M.D.s in charge of the program, for much the same reasons, I'll bet, that dictators use prisoners as block wardens and camp guards. Anyway, doctors are the managers of CPRO, so we poor foot soldiers who take care of patients had better listen, or else.

But it isn't easy. For example, I'll quote three paragraphs from a letter I received that outlined the ways CPRO's procedures have been altered:

"(1) Issues of quality having a significant impact on patient care or outcome will require a response by the physician of record.

"(2) Issues of quality which are deemed of lesser impact by the reviewing physician or reflect a difference of opinion of judgment having a lesser impact on patient care may be responded to by the physician of record or a physician assigned by the hospital to assume responsibility for replying to these issues.

"(3) Issues limited to quality of documentation in the record will be referred to the appropriate physician in the hospital for tracking. CPRO will also maintain its tracking file on these issues."

I've read this more than four times, written it once, reviewed it, and I still don't understand what my *Kommandant* is saying. Perhaps you can translate these paragraphs into English while I continue to sit at my desk, chin in hand, shaking my head in bewilderment. In my opinion, "impacting" and "tracking" are terms better suited to military games than to medical care.

In my part of the country, the most deprecatory thing you used to be able to say about a doctor was that he had married money. You've all heard the statements: "Of course old Doc Mergatroyd wouldn't go out at night on an emergency call—his wife is worth a bundle." Or "You could afford to write a trashy newspaper column, too, if your wife had dough." Not having married money, I'm not intimidated by such small-town sniping.

In my view, one of the worst things you can say about a doctor today is that he works for the government, because that indicates he no longer cares about patients and what it means to be sick.

If Aunt Zelda's $7,516.18 hospital bill is refused by a CPRO doctor, it wouldn't be any more right or acceptable than if it were turned down by a state accountant with a green eyeshade. We're dealing with people, dammit, and I get burned up when some physician I've never met tells me what to do, just because he's on the government payroll and happens to have the same medical degree I do.

The final sentence of the CPRO missive I quoted above is a beaut: "Your continued input is requested."

If I had a choice, I'd input that letter right back where it came from. As a physician of record, I'd impact that doctor until his own computer couldn't track him. I'd take his "timeframes," his "clarifying comments," his "prescribed procedures" and...

THE MALPRACTICE LOTTERY

We seem increasingly to be living in the Lottery Generation. State lotteries routinely give away millions of dollars to wonderfully ordinary citizens who plunk down a buck or two and pick a few numbers. Later, on the evening news, we are treated to the spectacle of elevator operators and factory workers who win more money than a corporate raider. These lucky winners are set for life; they can kiss their jobs goodbye, purchase a Rolls and move to air-conditioned splendor in the Sunbelt. We all envy them.

Lotteries are probably harmless. They reward the common man without respect to age, race, sex or religion. They swell the states' coffers; they provide jobs. More important, they provide hope.

Nevertheless, I'm concerned that the Lottery Mentality—

the belief that everyone deserves a big payoff on very little investment—may be one explanation for the current malpractice disaster that continues to undermine the day-by-day service given by doctors. From what I read, and in talking to colleagues, I am beginning to perceive that increasing numbers of patients are viewing medical care as a lottery, with financial rewards—not health—as the goal. To the practicing physician and surgeon, each patient is becoming a potential liability, rather than a person who needs help. Soon, the public is going to realize that this is not the way the system of health care will work most effectively.

A few years ago, while taking a patient's medical history, I asked a routine question about how many children he had. "I had four," he replied. "We lost one at two years of age." "How did that happen?" I inquired. "Well," he said, "the doctor gave her a diphtheria shot and she died." "That's awful," I sympathized; "did you sue?" "Hell, no!" he exclaimed. "The doc did the best he could. It was just one of those things."

I don't want to return to the days when normal two-year-olds were at greater risk of dying from immunization injections, nor am I suggesting that patients who are injured by doctors should not attempt to receive legal recompense. However, the pendulum has swung right off the clock. The goose that lays golden malpractice awards is on the way to being cooked.

Some doctors are now required to pay up to $100,000 a year in malpractice premiums. Of course, they pass on the overhead to patients, causing further escalation of medical costs. Many experts predict that, before long, malpractice insurance may simply dry up; it may not be available at any fee. Then doctors will have to make agonizing decisions about whether or not they can afford to practice medicine at all. Society, the consumer and the patient will all suffer.

There is a sad truth in my patient's statement that "it was just one of those things." Life itself is brimming with unpredictabilities; medications are risky; surgery is dangerous.

You may be interested to look at workmen's compensation benefits. In my state, the loss of a hand is "worth" $78,120; a finger, $8,060 to $16,740; one eye, $72,850; hearing in both ears, $48,360. That's what a worker is paid if he or she is seriously injured, in any of a variety of ways, on the job. However, if the person loses an appendage or sight or hearing because of a medical mishap, the damages are likely to be in the millions of dollars.

We need some consistency here. The loss of a leg in a mill accident is just as tragic and disabling as loss of a limb from a surgical mistake, yet it is compensated at far less than its medical counterpart. Doctors may feel a need to "act perfect" and not acknowledge their mistakes because to do otherwise would be to invite calamitous lawsuits.

Some patients—indeed, some judges—look on malpractice as a lottery. In our litigious society, ordinary dangers become someone's fault. An unpleasant outcome, even a temporary one, is rarely considered to be "one of those things."

I am not one who whines about the problems doctors have. However, I think the public must realize the extent to which malpractice concerns and frivolous suits are affecting every practicing doctor—the really good ones, too. If patients cannot bring themselves to adopt a less financially oriented outlook, medical care as we know it will deteriorate into what has already been called "defensive medicine": the preoccupation with protecting one's flanks in preference to treating and healing the needy. Medical care must not degenerate into a lottery. Under such an arrangement, for every winner there are a lot of losers. And it is truly the patients who will lose in a medical lottery system.

THE
HIGH-TECH
FUTURE

❖

There's a new medical test available that, in the next few years, probably will supersede most of the current X-ray high tech, including the CAT scan—unless that scanner has nine lives.

The test is called Magnetic Resonance Imaging (MRI). It's very expensive at present, so it's available in only a few of the larger hospitals and in selected radiologists' offices. But it's a breakthrough, no doubt. Because you'll be hearing more about it, you might be interested in knowing how it works.

Everything in the world is composed of atoms. These atoms are made up of several elementary charged particles, one of which is called a proton. In their natural state, protons are minuscule spinning balls that swirl around the nucleus of each atom. Protons are indescribably small, and in the total scheme of things, they don't amount to much. However, they have one fascinating attribute: when placed in a strong magnetic field and bombarded by high-frequency radio waves, they become "excited" and soak up energy. They then behave like tiny magnets and adopt similar spinning and rotating characteristics, orienting in unison like little soldiers on parade. Once random protons are twirling in step, they give off some of the energy they've picked up.

This energy, in the form of radio signals, can be measured, recorded and, through a complex series of computerized functions, made into pictures. Since hydrogen is the most common atom in the body, MRI machines actually are mapping the concentration of hydrogen protons in tissues. Dense, proton-rich structures produce different patterns than do less-dense proton-poor substances.

The extraordinary result of this complicated imaging technique is a photograph very much like an X-ray film but far more detailed. This miracle is accomplished without the use of injections or potentially lethal radiation. It's basically a pictorial means of quantifying energy that exists in the components of atoms themselves.

Of course, the machinery used in this testing is extremely sophisticated, and people who operate it must undergo extensive training. The electromagnet alone is strong enough to suck the fillings out of your teeth if they were magnetic. The amount of pull, far exceeding the magnetic force of the earth itself, is about eight times more powerful than that created by the giant magnets that pick up derelict cars in junkyards.

Despite this awesome power, there is no known danger to humans from either the magnet or the radio waves—no disruption of DNA, no requirement to limit exposure, no risk of allergic reaction, no depression of blood-forming organs or reproductive tissue.

I'm sure that many years will elapse before MRI is generally available to the public in doctors' offices and community hospitals. However, this test does prove that our own physicists, when given enough motivation, can come up with superlative new modalities of medical investigation.

X rays are dangerous, despite some doctors' patronizing reassurances to the contrary. I suppose that, as time progresses, some MRI hazards will be identified. Even so, we have the knowledge to continue pushing back frontiers of the new and different. If there's anything exciting about medicine of the future, frontier wrangling is it.

NO TURNING BACK

❖

In 1818 Mary Shelley published her classical horror story about the Frankenstein monster, a creature composed of bodies robbed from graves, crudely sewn together and given life by high-voltage electricity administered by a crazed scientist living in a dark castle. Mary Shelley herself characterized the novel as a "ghost story." It was pure fantasy. No responsible person in the early 1800s considered the story of Dr. Frankenstein's experiment to have a shred of truth or value outside the world of fiction.

Today, more than a century and a half later, doctors are using, as a matter of routine, electronic heart pacemakers, brain grafts, plastic hearts, lungs and kidneys from cadavers, synthetic arteries, artificial limbs and transplanted human organs. Surgeons can now sew back on completely severed appendages, and the patient can achieve almost full use of the reconstructed part. A short while ago, the world was thrilled by the birth of a baby who had been conceived outside her mother's body; the procedure is almost commonplace now. Are we one up on Dr. Frankenstein? Mary Shelley would probably be astounded by the current work in the field of genetic engineering, called recombinant-DNA research, or "cloning."

Long the mainstay of science fiction, cloning refers to the development of an adult organism from a single cell grown in the laboratory. Each of us carries in each of our cells the necessary genetic information to make a whole living being. However, because of natural restraints within the body, most of our cells remain specialized: a skin cell continues to be a skin cell, a muscle cell divides to make more muscle cells, and so forth. For many years, scientists have been attempting to tease certain cells into branching out and becoming something new. In 1980, this became a reality. In the laboratory, under artificial conditions, separate cells from a mouse were treated to result in the growth of three identical adult mice.

The potential consequences of this act are enormous. Scientists are now developing methods by which, in theory, humans can be nonsexually replicated. The end result could be an almost infinite number of identical beings all grown from the same single cell. No wonder cloning has captured the imagination of nonscientists as well as professionals.

The concept of genetic engineering seems terrifying; we are tampering with the stuff of life itself, reducing people to the level of mass-reproduced look-alike items, creating new lifeforms. Although we are many years from achieving the "manufacture" of a human form from an adult cell, certain citizens' lobbies and congressmen have demanded—and succeeded in obtaining—a moratorium on cloning research. People are worried that cloning, now in its infancy, may grow into a Frankenstein monster and veer out of control. Even fertilization of human eggs outside the body is seen as threat.

I suggest that it is no answer to return to the simple life of a pretechnological age. Mammalian cloning is inevitable. Instead of looking the other way or hiding under the bedclothes, we had better start thinking about and dealing with the moral and legal questions raised by scientific discoveries. A stupendous amount of good could accrue from cloning research: knowledge about birth defects, inherited diseases, cancer, wound healing and organ regeneration. An educated public, willing to wrestle with the ethical problems of cloning, is far more preferable than a broad ban fostered by uninformed public opinion. A climate of rational open-mindedness is a must.

Because of its delicate and intricate nature, cloning is not the kind of activity carried out by maniacal scientists in musty attics, Gothic castles or moldy basement laboratories. Rather, it lends itself to continued public scrutiny and regulation by responsible researchers. Today's scientists may be on the verge of making discoveries that will extend our lives as well as improve the quality of our existence. Isn't it fascinating to be a front-row observer of this astonishing revolution?

Twentieth-century technology has propelled us, willy-nilly, into a new, bewildering science-fiction world. And nowhere have I been reminded more of this difficult transition than in the Rios case, an extreme example of the alarming implications of one new advance.

For reasons unclear to me, American parents Mario and Elsa Rios decided to have a family in a particularly unique manner. In Australia, two of Elsa's ova were fertilized, in vitro, outside her body. The embryos were frozen in liquid nitrogen in states of suspended animation. Two years later, the millionaire parents died in a plane crash in Chile. Now the fate of the embryos—which were set aside for future implantation—is in doubt. There are no parents or guardians. The three-day-old embryos became "orphans." If the legal problems of inheritance are a lawyer's nightmare, the moral dilemmas of the case may be even more substantial.

A nine-member ethics committee of Queen Victoria Hospital in Melbourne apparently recommended destroying the embryos, but there was such a public outcry against this "solution" that the Australian authorities are, at the time of this writing, unsure of how to proceed.

Evidently, there are 250 frozen embryos at Queen Victoria Hospital alone. If that number reflects in any way the world population of frozen embryos, we are dealing with a considerable constituency whose legal status has yet to be determined.

I am not knowledgeable about how fertilized ova are frozen and stored. But you don't have to be an expert to begin wondering about the issues raised by the process. I'd always assumed that when parents started a family, they would want to hold the baby, see it, at least know that it is growing and thriving. Presumably, some parents who conceive children in vitro expect a surrogate mother to come along, in whom the embryo can be implanted.

The presence of hundreds of frozen, motherless embryos makes me speculate about whether the world is inexplicably short of mothers or whether procreation is taking a different tack—toward furnishing an almost endless supply of tiny human beings upon which to experiment. I'm not wildly enthusiastic about the prospect of a class of citizens raised for this purpose. I'd always assumed white rats were preferable.

The thirty childless couples who offered to adopt the Rios "orphans" no doubt announced their candidacies for purely humanitarian reasons. But the fact that Mr. and Mrs. Rios left a bundle of money thrust them into a bizarre and inhumane lottery with winner take all. Surely, the price is right.

For couples unable to bear children, legitimate in-vitro fertilization is clearly a heaven-sent miracle. But there is a troublesome aspect to this procedure. Maybe we ought to back off a bit, think things through and deal with the ethical problems until there are sufficient numbers of suitable, warm-blooded women willing to sign on the dotted line, ready to commit to limited nine-month maternities.

I should note that a British ethics committee recently condemned the concept of surrogate motherhood. In addition, Australian scientists are now talking about experimenting on "spare embryos" up to fourteen days of age. I don't believe that, as a race, we can afford "spare embryos." If an ovum is fertilized, the product of that union ought to be guaranteed a parent, and the fertilization shouldn't take place unless that parent is immediately available.

You see, if scientists can successfully store frozen embryos, what's to prevent them from developing techniques to nourish thawed embryos? Enable them to grow and develop? Raise them? Train them?

H. G. Wells and Aldous Huxley would have appreciated the possibilities.

THE BUBBLE AND ITS CONSEQUENCES

A few years ago, I described a baby boy in Texas who was born into—and was living in—an environment free of germs.

Doctors had predicted that because of an inherited genetic defect David would be born without immunity to disease. He would be unable to manufacture lymphoid tissue, the stuff lymph nodes are made of. It is in the lymph nodes that antibodies are manufactured, enabling normal people to arrest an infection literally before it gets started. David was thought to be utterly devoid of lymphoid tissue and, therefore, would have died of infection resulting from any one of the hundreds of bacterial types that normal babies are exposed to in the first few weeks of life.

After a completely germfree birth—prior to which the delivery room had been sealed and scrubbed for three consecutive days—David was placed inside a sterile plastic bubble. He lived in the bubble all his life.

He grew normally. The artificial environment was large enough for him to walk, which he did at eight months of age, and flexible enough so that doctors and attendants—through sealed arm holes—could feed him, touch him and treat almost any medical emergency, including fractures.

From a medical standpoint, the child's survival was miraculous. All his physical needs were taken care of. Psychiatrists studied the child and devoted long hours to his emotional development. He showed satisfactory intellectual progress.

Despite the medical marvels of the production, I wonder whether, in fact, David's doctors painted themselves into a corner. The child showed no evidence that he could ever acquire resistance to disease. Essentially, he had to remain in his plastic isolator, playing with aseptic toys and eating sterile food indefinitely. For twelve years, he spent his entire life sheltered within a plastic envelope. In 1977, NASA gave him a space suit, which enabled him to hug his mother and play for short periods in his backyard. Inside the house, he remained in his plastic bubble and attended school by telephone. In October 1983, in a desperate attempt to provide him with disease-fighting white blood cells, David received a bone-marrow transplant from his fifteen-year-old sister. The transplant was not successful. The following February, David was removed from his bubble for treatment of dehydration resulting from diarrhea and vomiting. On that day, he kissed his mother for the first time. Once out of his artificial environment, he could never return to it. A few days later, in critical condition, David knew he was dying and asked the doctors to let him "go home." His wish was granted.

The scientific miracles that allowed David to survive for twelve years are real; these spin-offs of space-age technology will undoubtedly be used in the future to help other immune-deficient children. David's doctors are obviously sensitive and dedicated professionals. His parents and sister must be unusually caring and courageous people. David himself was a very special human being.

The story of this gallant child raises important questions about, among other issues, the quality of his life. Once scientists decide to keep someone alive, there is a responsibility to the patient that may transcend the purely physical act of prolonged life. In David's case, how could the doctors provide for human touch and contact as he developed? How long can a person survive in such an environment without showing signs of emotional deprivation? Are the expense and anguish worth the end result? Most important: Was it fair to David?

There are some thinkers who believe we are closer to a *Brave New World* existence than we care to admit. More than a decade ago, David's parents made a decision, a very personal decision with far-reaching consequences. Other parents, given the option, might have made another decision. One fact is clear: The moral aspects of scientific advances are quite separate from the purely technical advances. And this dichotomy is as apparent in the case of an immunologically deficient boy in a bubble as it is in cases of abortion, euthanasia for the aged, organ transplantation and artificial insemination: problems with which twentieth-century man must cope using an eighteenth-century moral foundation.

We all lost a friend when David died. Each of us is a better person because of him. In each of us is the seed of strength that this remarkable youngster displayed daily. His courage and spirit, his will and perseverance, are gifts he gave us by example. I'm truly sorry we lost him.

The newspapers said he wanted to walk barefoot in the grass. He never did. But I am confident that his legacy was an astounding gift. Perhaps he will give strength to the weak, confidence to the sick, and hope to all of us. For me, David's death is an abiding reminder of the value of life. Children are exceptional and marvelous; sick children are even more exceptional.

I won't forget David, nor, I suspect, will anyone who knew of him and his tremendous battle for life.

CHAPTER 14

SOME
PATHS
TO
GOOD
MEDICINE

A CODE OF MEDICAL PRACTICE

❖

Things seem to have reached a pretty sorry state of affairs for the medical profession in some, if not all, parts of the country. Apparently the situation has deteriorated to the point where some consumers "aren't going to take it anymore"; they have begun to organize into quasi-political bodies in order to educate doctors in how to be human. One such group, the People's Medical Society in Emmaus, Pennsylvania, has developed a Code of Practice. The society's shortened name, PMS, bears no relation to premenstrual syndrome (the other PMS), but it is surely going to be a pain and a discomfort for many M.D.s. Those physicians who sign the code will be included in a national directory that will be available to PMS members—a sort of medical fifth column, as it were.

When I read through the code, I experienced a pang of sadness. It seems humiliating for doctors to have to be reminded of proper behavior that I've always assumed was an axiom of the profession. But that's the way it is. A lot of patients are fed up to here with doctors' antics. Perhaps this document will serve to remind us that in our hell-bent-for-leather pursuit of the scientific Grail, we may, in the process, be sacrificing equally important principles of humanism.

Many physicians are surprised at the vehemence of the PMS position, because, for these doctors, the code has been an unspoken and integral part of their life's work. These are not the healers who are indicted by the People's Medical Society. Yet the mere existence of a Code of Practice reflects a militant acknowledgment that there are doctors out there who seem to have forgotten what doctoring is all about.

Here is the Code of Practice, along with my editorial comments:

"1. I will post or provide a printed schedule of my fees for office visits, procedures, testing and surgery, and provide itemized bills." This seems fairly straightforward. I agree that the courteous physician should, in some manner, indicate the basis for his fee schedule. Printed or posted material may not be the most practical way of accomplishing this goal, however. To a large extent, fees are flexible and may be mightily influenced by time spent on complicated cases as well as by what is known among competitive platform divers as "degree of difficulty." For example, I am going to charge more for treating a patient with a complex illness or an unstable heart attack than I would for a session of less demanding activity like counseling. Nonetheless, most doctors can give a fairly accurate ball-park figure in advance of the service; this is an appropriate principle to follow. Many M.D.s feel awkward discussing fees with patients. We're not trained in this activity; we sort of have to pick it up in the wild, after we enter practice. Fortunately, most doctors have the capacity to learn new behavior, and there is nothing to equal an informed patient for giving continuing medical education to the physician.

"2. I will provide certain hours each week when I will be available for nonemergency telephone consultations." This is child's play for the pediatricians, but it is somewhat of an anachronism for those of us who treat adults. My telephone rings all day. If I'm not busy, I talk to patients; if I'm occupied, I'll return the call. I have never understood doctors who insulate themselves from telephone calls. The phone is often a nuisance, but it is a lifeline for patients. Without it, our practices would wither; we would not be able to conduct our business. The doctor who is not available at reasonable times ought to consider another line of work. You can bet that telephone calls from stockbrokers, attorneys, colleagues and that cute divorcée down the street are promptly tended to. Why not offer the same courtesy to patients?

This raises another issue: Doctors who charge for routine telephone consultations. Yes, I know it's done, but as a practice it seems to be one more manifestation of money-grubbing and medical arrogance. Lawyers are the only other professionals I know who make a point of charging for telephone calls. Do we doctors really want to mimic the legal guild? No, let's keep complimentary, open lines of communication. Life is tough enough for ill patients without doctors nickel-and-diming them to death.

"3. I will schedule appointments to allow necessary time to see you with minimal waiting. I will promptly return test results to you and phone calls." Sounds reasonable, but it's sometimes as hard for a doctor to stay on schedule as it is for him to trade in his BMW for a Ford Escort. It's a sign of affluence to have a full waiting room, and, unhappily, many patients still cling to the baroque notion that all seemingly busy doctors are successful and brilliant. It isn't so. The physician with the overflowing waiting room may be just plain inefficient or he may have orchestrated his office hours to capitalize on the rush. In the event that the doctor is held up by a bona fide emergency, his secretary could reschedule appointments—but the doctor may not bother to notify her. A captive audience of needful office patients is an almost insurmountable temptation. The doctor convinces himself he must be good or else patients wouldn't wait an interminable time to see him. This is straight ego gratification.

"4. I will allow and encourage you to bring a friend or relative into the examining room with you." I'm not in favor of this position unless the patient is under ten years of age. Most adults I know are not eager to bare themselves to a curious bystander, particularly if the examination involves breasts, reproductive tract or lower intestine. In the event, however, that a patient requests that a spouse or relative be present, I honor the request. For appropriate female examinations, the prudent physician would want to have a nurse or woman assistant present. Finally, I do not encourage family observation of nonpediatric treatment. This experience can be unpleasant, the third person often gets in the way, and the situation can be embarrassing for the patient. In my opinion, the examining room is reserved for adult patient, doctor and other trained professionals. These comments hold for the examing room only; I encourage patients to bring friends and family into the consulting room for discussion.

"5. I will facilitate your getting your medical and hospital records, and will provide you with copies of your test results." On the surface, this appears to be a reasonable agreement, but there are problems. Medical records are really for the doctor's own use. We frequently use medical abbreviations and terms that are unintelligible to the layman. I once indicated on a hospital record of an overweight young man that he was "obese," the accepted medical term for someone with excessive body weight. When the hospital released the record to him for insurance purposes, he was incensed at being labeled "obese." He spent many acrimonious minutes on the telephone insisting that I had no right to characterize him in such a way although he admitted he was "slightly overweight." Medical records are not written to be complimentary to patients; the records are supposed to contain factual data that provide an accurate assessment of a person's physical and mental condition, what treatment was administered and its outcome.

My reluctance to hand over medical records does not mean I endorse secrecy. On the contrary, I make an effort to discuss fully with patients their medical problems. In addition, I take special pains to forward medical records to other doctors, on request, so that they can have the benefit of my evaluation. In the main, I oppose the recommendation that office and hospital records be released to an individual patient. If such a policy were to become widely accepted, I fear the quality and honesty of medical records might be compromised. In our computer-oriented society, there is already too free a flow of privileged information. Patients have a right to a coherent, detailed and understandable synopsis of their conditions, but my records stay in a locked cabinet for my use and will not be distributed unless I am legally required to do so or am asked to transfer these records to another physician.

"6. I will let you know your prognosis, including whether your condition is terminal or will cause disability or pain, and will explain why I believe further diagnostic activity or treatment is necessary." Bravo! I hope we are at last beginning to emerge from the mythical and secret cultishness of organized medicine. I might add, however, that not all patients wish to be told the exact nature and prognosis of their illnesses. It is cruel for an inconsiderate physician to force this information on patients who may be unready or unwilling to hear it. Much of the vanishing "art" of medicine involves making daily judgments about how much and in what form patients can best be educated about their diseases. If asked a specific question, I reply honestly. Nevertheless, that answer may require many variations and can take many days of reaffirmation to set in. True, patients have a right to know their prognoses and disabilities, but each in his own way, in his own time and at his own pace. Certainly, the discussion of further diagnostic investigation is vital to good patient care, and it is here that the patient and doctor can work appropriately as a team.

"7. I will discuss diagnostic, treatment and medication options for your particular problem with you (including the option of no treatment) and describe in understandable terms the risk of each alternative, the chances of success, the possibility of pain, the effect on your functioning, the number of visits each would entail, and the cost of each alternative." This article sounds great, but if you're like me, after a second reading you'll appreciate how cumbersome it is. It's a bit like agreeing to predict who will be president in 1994. On the whole, doctors have a responsibility to explain things to patients and to obtain what is called "informed consent" before treatment begins. Again, there is a question of degree here, as well as the sheer ponderousness of explaining every detail. Furthermore, doctors, being human after all, are often notoriously inept at crystal-ball gazing. For example, if I see a patient with a hernia, I am not clairvoyant to the point where I can chart his future. The hernia may remain nothing more than an inconvenience for twenty years, so the cheapest solution is to let it alone. On the other hand, it could strangulate (become wedged) next week, tonight or on New Year's Eve; then surgery would be necessary. How could I, in my right mind, predict the surgical fee, possible complications, or number of postoperative visits? I'd sooner speculate on next year's weather. Perhaps my patient's hernia will require surgery at an inconvenient time, when he is on a fishing trip to the North Woods or has just come off a serious bout of pneumonia. Under these circumstances, surgery could be downright dangerous; the unpredictable could occur.

I believe the thrust of principle #7 is to ensure that every patient has access (and is entitled) to reasonable information upon which to make rational judgments. But, in my opinion, no doctor could possibly meet the written requirements of the article. A physician's discretion must count for something: good doctors are judicious and thorough, within reason, in discussing options with patients. Bad doctors? Well, you can't trust what they say anyhow.

"8. I will describe my qualifications to perform the proposed diagnostic measure or treatments." No comment. A doctor's training and qualifications ought to be an open book to any person he serves.

"9. I will let you know of organizations, support groups, and medical and lay publications that can assist you in understanding, monitoring and treating your problem." I would add "providing the sources are reputable."

Healing is big business now, and it seems as though everyone wants to get into the act. You don't have to be mentally gifted to appreciate that doctors earn comfortable livings. For an unqualified and unprincipled egocentric, the next logical question is "Why not me too?" The temptation is great, and masses of disgruntled patients, fed up with traditional medicine, are ripe for exploitation by con men (and women) who offer easy cures through quackery. Not all "organizations" are reputable, not all support groups are therapeutic, and not all publications are ethical. These objections notwithstanding, reputable paramedical resources can be enormously helpful and should be part of every physician's equipment.

"10. I will not proceed until you are satisfied that you understand the benefits and risks of each alternative and I have your agreement on a particular course of action." This is pretty standard procedure, in my experience. Of course, some doctors continue to intimidate patients by insisting that only the healers are qualified to decide how to handle a certain situation. For the most part, however, people nowadays don't go for these antique, high-handed tactics. I believe that more patients are rightfully demanding a say in questions relating to their disorders. I think this is a grand way to equalize the doctor-patient relation. The physician is, after all, a trained professional whom you have hired to fix something. He works for you. You are paying him for his service, and he has an obligation to include you in the decision-making process.

I suppose I am saddened by this Code of Practice because of its truths. It is saying: "Doctor, treat patients like people; be understanding, compassionate, considerate, fair, forthright, honest in your self-evaluation, and communicative." Many physicians embody these principles. They go about their active professional lives with skill and confidence, buoyed up by grateful patients; they experience the same fears, disappointments and insecurities that plague any sane adult. They don't ruminate about PMS and Codes for Practice because there was a time, not so long ago, when these attributes were taken for granted by every physician who entered the healing profession. What we're talking about here is an issue of manners and decency, two qualities that have become, it seems, in short supply on doctors' shelves. Medical courtesy is not about to be supplanted by the glories of high-tech science. It's humbling to be reminded that the public notices how we behave and sometimes folks out there don't like what they see.

ANNUAL EXAMINA- TIONS RECONSIDERED

Traditionally, the doctor's role has been to heal the sick. Recently, however, politicians and people in the news media have questioned this approach. These medically uninformed individuals have insisted that a doctor's primary responsibility is to provide "preventive" medical care. The public is unaware, perhaps, that physicians have always provided preventive care in the form of vaccinations, immunization and so forth. The type of preventive care for heart disease, cancer and other serious illnesses now demanded by naïve legislators is not scientifically or financially feasible at this time for a variety of reasons, the most important being that we simply do not know enough about these diseases to prevent them. Furthermore, medical tests are, for the most part, relatively crude and are usually helpful in only a broad sort of way. There is nothing magical about a medical examination. Rather, the approach is a practical, logical sequence involving the painstaking collection and identification of information—and the careful application of that information. Many doctors are concerned that the public has an unrealistic view of what physicians and medicine can do. And nowhere is this unrealistic belief more obvious than in the concept of the "annual physical checkup" or the so-called "executive work-up."

It has been common practice for thousands of healthy Americans to undergo annual examinations and be subjected to an endless series of expensive and sometimes dangerous tests to make sure "everything is all right." Certain well-informed and farsighted physicians are starting to question the usefulness of the annual checkup; many articles have appeared in the medical journals indicating that the annual physical examination serves no purpose except to provide considerable income for doctors and to accentuate, experts say, the already neurotic preoccupation that most Americans have with health.

Patients with known diseases under treatment should certainly be checked periodically at the discretion of their private physicians. But what about the healthy adult who has no symptoms? Several studies have shown that the percentage of these individuals who are found to have significant disease on routine examination is practically nil: something less than 1 percent. What about this small percentage; are these people helped? As a general rule, no. For example, there is absolutely no evidence to indicate that the early identification of diseases such as diabetes or arteriosclerotic heart disease and certain cancers makes a substantial difference in the eventual outcome.

There is no doubt that individuals with symptoms should be thoroughly evaluated and that patients under treatment or observation should be periodically examined and tested. But it has been said, with a great deal of truth, that the average American doctor often spends so much time examining healthy people that he has limited time to see sick patients. Furthermore, the cost of an annual checkup, which can run as high as $500, is often not covered by insurance and can be a real burden to a middle-income family whose members dutifully visit the doctor each year.

Proponents of the annual examination have agreed that although the yield of positive findings is small, the ritualistic search is justified when some unsuspected disease is discovered. Unfortunately, this is not the case. By the time a cancer, for instance, is discovered through our rather crude means, it is usually large enough (at least a half inch in diameter) to have spread. We know that the important factor in curing cancer is *not* how big it is or how long it has been present, but what kind of cancer it is. Scientists have documented that treatment is essentially the same whether a cancer is symptom-producing or discovered accidentally. Furthermore, early treatment rarely modifies the future of the cancer patient; a highly malignant growth usually spreads before it can be detected; a low-grade malignancy may not spread until the tumor has grown quite large and has caused symptoms. There are three notable exceptions to this rule: cancer of the cervix in females, some breast cancers and certain tumors of the large intestine. In one case, the Pap smear will usually detect early trouble; this test should be performed yearly on all sexually active women in the reproductive years. In the case of bowel and breast tumors, there is some evidence that early detection by a variety of means can lead to cure.

Diabetes, despite government proclamations to the contrary, is still a relatively mild condition in most instances. The person who develops diabetes in childhood has a much more severe form of the disease and usually requires insulin injections. The elderly adult who is found to have diabetes can frequently be treated with diet and weight reduction alone. There is striking evidence showing that in this type of adult diabetes, control of high blood sugar *in no way changes the course of the disease*. In fact, a recent controversial study indicated that certain forms of pill treatment may actually be *detrimental* and accelerate the development of heart disease in diabetics. Many doctors believe that if the diabetes is significant enough to require treatment, the patient will almost always have symptoms suggesting the diagnosis, which can then be confirmed by appropriate laboratory analyses.

Medical literature is replete with case reports of patients who have undergone thorough and extensive examination only to suffer fatal heart attacks upon leaving their doctors' offices. Again, this is understandable because our tests are as yet not sensitive enough to predict in all instances the presence of heart disease. However, proponents of the annual checkup persist in publicizing the totally unrealistic merits of the examination. Heart disease severe enough for treatment produces symptoms. A knowledgeable physician can, through careful questioning, pinpoint the trouble. But it is rare that a patient undergoing the ceremony of annual examination is discovered to have a serious heart condition that was unsuspected. Other forms of heart disease, such as congenital malformations, are usually picked up by the pediatrician during the (necessary) routine examinations of infants.

Arteriosclerosis, diabetes, most cancers and other serious illnesses are *not*, by current medical technology, preventable or cured by early detection. Nor will they be in the future by wholesale annual examinations of healthy adults. If doctors really believed that annual checkups were necessary and helpful, they themselves would undergo them. In truth, they don't, as a rule. Several experts have suggested that the American public would do far better being less concerned about health and more concerned about disease and its manifestations.

At present, it seems reasonable to adopt a middle-ground approach to annual health examinations. Patients with any persisting changes in their normal life patterns—for example, bowel changes, difficulty in breathing, pain, unexplained weight loss and fatigue—should definitely check with their physicians and undergo appropriate evaluation. Women in the reproductive years should have Pap tests and breast examinations. Infants and children should be examined periodically during their formative years. There is really no need for those healthy adults who are symptom-free and who want annual examinations to be subjected automatically to extensive and expensive laboratory investigation. A competent physician who takes a careful and detailed history and then performs a thorough examination (and selected laboratory tests as indicated) can tell as much as the impersonal doctor in a big medical center who orders multiple batteries of laboratory analyses in a shotgun approach. Healthy adults who choose to avoid annual checkups need not necessarily feel guilty. Life is more enjoyable when one does not constantly worry about imagined ills. However, the prudent healthy adult will probably want to adhere to this guideline: one complete examination in the twenties, one in the thirties, one in the forties, examination every three to five years in the fifties, annually thereafter. Doctors are always prepared to help cure disease and should be consulted when appropriate. But a good physician, along with recognizing his own weaknesses and strengths, must also recognize how incredibly limited scientific medicine is at the present time. It is his or her responsibility to share this realization with his patients.

Finally, the obsession with laboratory tests and so-called "routine" checkups has resulted in a new disease: the Ulysses syndrome. The condition has been reported in the *Journal of the American Medical Association*: "The Ulysses syndrome is a complex of mental and physical disorders which follows the discovery of a false-positive result in the course of routine laboratory screening. Because a physician worth his diagnostic salt would hardly pass up the challenge of such a result, he pursues the investigation 'just to make sure.' This pursuit may lead to other false-positives which in turn provoke further investigations, until after a long journey through investigative adventures—some physically, mentally and financially traumatic— the patient finally returns to the point of departure, just as Ulysses to Ithaca after twenty years of odyssey.

"[One author] ascribes the Ulysses syndrome to mischievous investigations promoted by mass screening projects and insurance examinations, to neurotic patient reactions, to the physician's hope of serendipitous discovery, to retention of outdated tests on standard laboratory forms, and to the doctor's uncritical interpretation of laboratory reports. A physician, aware that about 5 percent of normal people will have laboratory values outside the laboratory ranges of normality and thus will be false-positive, should be able to restrain his zeal for investigative pursuits."

Many physicians are reappraising traditional beliefs regarding ritualistic annual physical examinations of healthy adults. Pediatricians too are re-evaluating the concept of frequent examinations for children. For years the medical profession has encouraged frequent checkups by doctors as a way of preventing and detecting serious illness. Within the pediatric age group, this has taken the form of four-to-six week examinations during the first year of life and yearly checkups thereafter. There is no question that this has led to more infants receiving immunizations and being protected against serious diseases such as polio, diphtheria, tetanus, pertussis, measles and rubella. Likewise, serious congenital defects have been recognized and treated earlier and more effectively.

The purpose of such examinations extends beyond immunization and detection of abnormalities. Maintaining health and preventing future problems are equally important goals. These include monitoring physical growth, assessing intellectual development, counseling in the areas of minor problems of normal infants (such as diet, behavior, sleep, toilet training and temper tantrums), and preventing accidental injury and serious problems of an emotional nature. To a great extent, these goals are achieved in affluent urban and surburban communities, but inadequate immunizations and routine medical care are frequently the rule in poorer rural and urban areas. As in the case of yearly physical exams for adults, pediatricians have traditionally and uncritically accepted the necessity of four-to-six-week evaluations for the infant. Recently, there has been some serious questioning and study of the need for such frequent visits. In addition, some pediatricians are wondering whether the physician needs to be the one who performs these exams. Typically, a pediatrician spends more than 50 percent of his working day caring for basically healthy children. Many children with physical, emotional or learning problems may not get needed attention because of constraints on the physician's time. Furthermore, the cost of routine exams may prevent a significant number of children from getting any care, except during acute illness.

There is good evidence to suggest that an infant need be seen for well-child exams only four to six times during the first year of life. From one to seven years of age, an annual exam is adequate. For the healthy school-age child, complete exams every two to three years have been shown to be quite satisfactory. The yearly school physical (characterized by the routine passing of the stethoscope over the bare chests of the students as they pass by the school doctor) has a value approaching zero. Cursory exams may result in overwrought parents who rush their children to the family doctor because of an innocent heart murmur or earwax. However, there is no question that hearing and vision screening (usually performed by a nurse) is quite important in this age group.

The biggest problems in the school-age child are not primarily physical (except for vision, hearing and dental) but are in the learning and guidance areas. To evaluate such problems takes time and the combined efforts of physicians, educators and psychologists in the school system. Communities that have begun to use their school physicians as consultants for children's problems have made considerable headway in recognizing and assisting the child who is having trouble—and perhaps even preventing the youngster from "turning school off" in the fourth or fifth grade.

The role of the pediatric nurse or pediatric nurse associate (a nurse who is a specialist in child health care) has become increasingly important over the past few years, both in the care of the infant and of the school-age child. A nurse's ability to perform physical exams, detect abnormalities, and counsel on child development and behavior is considered by many pediatricians to be on a par with their own. The fact that many of these nurses are themselves mothers who have been through the day-to-day experience of raising children makes them even more valuable resources. The association of the pediatric nurse practitioner with the physician has enabled the doctor to spend more time with the child who has specific problems.

The annual exam would itself profit from an objective examination by doctors and patients alike, who have for too long gone through the motions routinely year after year.

A COLLEAGUE'S PROVOCATIVE POSITION

❖

The current trend in this country to ensure good health threatens to immerse doctors in a morass of false expectations. Doctors are being expected to promise what they cannot deliver. In the *New England Journal of Medicine*, Dr. Mike Oppenheim wrote a thought-provoking article that, understandably, received no press coverage. He stated what people don't like to hear: namely, that doctors are trained to heal the sick; that is what they like to do and it's what they do best. He convincingly argued that longer lives and a healthier population are concerns best left to nonmedical personnel—teachers, for example. I would like to share with you some of his thoughts. Although I am taking his statements out of context, I'll make every effort to present his case fairly.

"The role of the American physician has changed over the past generation. The doctor seems to be taking responsibility for everyone all the time. People expect medical attention even when they feel fine. A healthy person who asked a British general practitioner for a complete physical would either be treated as a hypochondriac or shooed out of the office.

"Treating disease is not very efficient, but that is what doctors do. The public may protest, insisting that they want more than bandages and drugs. Most are probably unaware of what they really want from a doctor until they get a bellyache, then they know. [They] want a healer.

"A sick patient may object to the doctor's bill, but at least patients know what they are paying for. People who feel fine have to strain to pay health insurance, and may wonder what they are getting for the money.

"Doctors and hospitals soak up billions of dollars each year, and in the end they do not deliver much health. Heart disease and cancer are still our major killers, and no dramatic changes are in the works. Smokers smoke. People continue to eat poorly, behave stupidly, and die too soon.

"Keeping people healthy is important. To a limited extent, it is even feasible, but giving the job to doctors is foolish. A vigorous effort at health education would be a superb way to help Americans live longer.

"Research over the past decade makes it clear that only a handful of hidden, treatable diseases exists: hypertension, cervical cancer, glaucoma and perhaps bowel cancer. There is more to a complete physical [exam] than the physical itself. Patients do not complain when I decide not to do a rectal examination, but if I fail to include 'tests' I hear about it. In fact, no blood test or X-ray study performed regularly in a person who feels well is useful in detecting hidden, treatable disease. Health maintenance requires only a modest amount of skill. A screening examination is a collection of simple tests done over and over again. A nurse or trained layman can perform the useful part of a physical examination."

Dr. Oppenheim concluded his article by pointing out that a true breakthrough in health care will probably come only if the government subsidizes a program to educate the public, not just to pay medical bills. "These teams would travel through schools, offices, factories, and neighborhoods, checking blood pressures and doing Pap smears, breast examinations, and any other screening test that could pick up early signs of treatable disease. Smokers and unsafe drivers would be mercilessly harassed." A media blitz would be necessary.

Whether or not you agree with Dr. Oppenheim's position, you must admit it is provocative. Under his system, people would be educated about health and how to maintain it. Doctors would then be left free to treat illness, a role M.D.s are trained to perform and perform well. Health maintenance would become the responsibility of each citizen; doctors would, perhaps, no longer be blamed because they seem to promise goals that are unrealistic.

ON
HOUSE
CALLS

❖

I am fortunate to practice medicine in a part of the world where most doctors seem to have their patients' best interests as a primary concern. Perhaps that is an advantage of living in the country. For example, to my knowledge, all the doctors on the staff of our community hospital make house calls. What? Oh, you know, when the doctor calls on sick patients at home. Even surgeons here do it. And—hold on to your seat belt—so does our part-time dermatologist from Manhattan. Whatever is in the rural air must be catching.

To say that we are bucking a national trend is like pointing out that birds sing in the morning. It's obvious. Yet, so far the sky hasn't fallen because we choose to be quaintly old-fashioned.

In what passes for modern medicine in many parts of the nation, the house call is no longer in vogue. Like the zoot suit, the hoola-hoop and the wooden tennis racket, it is passé. Finito. A bit of nostalgia like the Tom Mix whistling ring. However, if you ask me, doctors who refuse to make house calls are missing a lot. So are their patients.

When Grandpa has a fever of 104 degrees and is delirious to the point of thinking he is Fred Flintstone, it's your problem, madam. If your child is so sick he cannot raise his head from the pillow, just sponge him down and drive him in sub-zero cold at 3 A.M. to your nearest emergency room. If, elderly person, your arthritis or heart failure prevents you from walking to the bathroom, so what? Hire a taxi and get to the office somehow or other.

"I don't make house calls because I couldn't possibly see patients at home in a setting where I lack the armamentarium of modern laboratory and X-ray equipment needed to maximize

the impact of health-care maintenance." Armamentarium? Lab
tests? What is this guy saying? I'll translate: pick your favorite.

The doctor can't be bothered.

It is not convenient for the doctor to come to your house.

The doctor can see six patients an hour in the office for
$150 and not have to fight sleet and traffic for a measly fifty
bucks.

The doctor would prefer to plant his ample buttocks on the
seat of his leather Gucci chair and wait in a comfy office for
sick people to come to him.

The doctor is so uncertain of his clinical judgment that he
wouldn't dream of diagnosing a house case, where he would
have to trust his hands, ears and eyes—the basic medical tools—
to arrive at a conclusion and give treatment.

The doctor is too important a life force to accede to the
demands of the infirm.

The doctor is a specialist and limits his practice to specific
organs, not people.

Of course this is an exaggeration—I think. The many doctors
who continue to make house calls are perfectly aware of the
services they provide, and they enjoy it. What are their reasons?

To begin with, house calls enable the physician to see firsthand what is going on at home. What's in the kitchen? Is nutritious food available? What is in the medicine cabinet? Lots
of surprises there, sometimes. Who is taking care of Aunt Maude?
Is there supervision of the children? Nursing help and proper
equipment? Is it a happy-feeling home? Depressing? Desperate?
Who lives there and under what circumstances?

Second, house calls may be cheaper for patients. In our
present climate of concern about excessive medical costs, I
believe it makes sense to diagnose and treat straightforward
problems at home. If the patient has to be transported to the
doctor's office or the hospital, there is added cost for family
members who may lose time from work, and hidden costs for
volunteer ambulance services. Heaven forbid the family should
have to use a commercial ambulance—they're useful but very
expensive. On top of transportation fees, patients seen in hos-

pital emergency rooms are forced to pay hospital charges plus the cost of (largely unnecessary) laboratory tests.

Third, sick patients are already uncomfortable enough without having to sit... and sit... and sit in unfamiliar waiting rooms. Nothing evokes as much sympathy as a young child, burning up with fever, waiting while more (or less) needy patients are being evaluated. In addition, ill patients are often contagious. It's hard to avoid getting sick when you have been sneezed at all afternoon in a waiting room.

Last, the house call is a convenience to the sick. The elderly, particularly on icy winter days, may find traveling to be an excruciating experience. Most medical problems can be resolved, by an average physician, at home—without the need of fancy gadgets or expensive medical toys. If hospitalization is required, the doctor is in an excellent position to coordinate early transport to the hospital and the initiation of diagnostic evaluation and treatment. House calls are a service that benefits both patient and doctor. Ask your physician if, when he is ill, he wouldn't prefer house care. Most doctors would; they have no more interest in traveling under these circumstances than you do.

Often the doctor who disdains making house calls is the first person to ask for one from a colleague—and then complain if he is charged. In my opinion, family doctors (general doctors, internists and primary-care physicians) owe patients the courtesy of house calls when necessary. If your physician refuses to make house calls, ask him why. If his reasons aren't sound, inquire as to the purpose of his brand-new expensive car and whether such a magnificent machine couldn't be put to better use than conspicuous consumption.

Modern medicine doesn't require that we give up time-proved services that are appreciated by patients under our care. Our job—I believe—is to help the sick, not to distance ourselves from them.

Informed consumers can bring about change. Find a doctor when you are healthy, not ill. Adopt a get-tough attitude. It works.

HEROES

❖

I am asked on occasion to name the real giants of medicine, the shakers, the clinicians who have enormous impact on doctors-in-training. For some reason, I am becoming less able to compile a list. I know there are remarkably skillful physicians in most of our finest medical schools and hospitals; many of these men and women would qualify as super docs. I am certain that my own ignorance of these special doctors' identities may interfere with the chore of establishing a reference guide of living medical giants. After all, the Gutmachers, Goldsmiths, Friedbergs, Loebs and Crohns, of my own training years, are dead and survive only as dog-eared memories for those of us who knew them.

However, I don't believe that my present lack of sophistication is the major determinant of my inability to categorize. Something in the medical world has changed and that change is not subtle.

The old clinicians, the professors we knew and looked up to, exhibited qualities that appear to be out of fashion today. These extraordinary doctors, like those before them, had great presence. They used their experience, judgment and phenomenal knowledge to diagnose an astounding array of ailments. They had charm, understanding and self-discipline. They were, at times, ferocious in their own gentle ways. They expected intellectual honesty in themselves and in others. As students and new doctors, we were terrified of them. But, at the same time, we were drawn to them because of their greatness.

They were never rude to patients. They were compassionate and understood the *meaning* of disease and discomfort; the meaning to each patient as a unique individual. In addition to dealing with difficult diseases, they helped patients cope with fear, hopelessness and loneliness.

Although they used laboratory values as tools, they never became servants to machines. They showed perspective. They taught by example and demanded loyalty to the sheer beauty of intellectualism and scientific thought. Their own personal lives may have been in disorder—we never cared and never asked. They were committed to the conviction that what they had could achieve meaning only by being given and shared.

I don't know if medical giants exist today. Like a civilized breed of mutants, they seem to have become extinct, leaving new forms of less-superlative beings in our barbarous world.

Yet, in retrospect, many of their qualities seem to linger in the most unlikely places: everyday Clark Kent physicians who carry on the honorable traditions of the healing profession, without the recognition and appreciation of anyone other than their own patients.

You know them. The doctor who makes house calls at 2 A.M. and then waives the bill. The physician who does not view death as an enemy in a suffering, terminally ill patient. The M.D. who will talk, explain, listen, understand, sympathize, be human. The healer who is not afraid to say "I don't know," who recognizes that he is fallible, but does his damndest to avoid making mistakes. The principled physician whose loyalties are to his patient, instead of to an old-boy network, his stock portfolio, or a hospital administration.

Come to think of it, there are such physicians out there. They're usually not rich; they just do their jobs because they obtain satisfaction and pleasure from serving those in need. These M.D.s are the new heroes of medicine. They are the resource that can save a profession. In their own quiet ways, they are unpublicized superstars. They live among us. They are the future. They're too numerous to list.

ABOUT THE AUTHOR

Dr. Peter Gott's medical column appears in more than 400 newspapers nationwide seven days a week. An independent survey has found him to be the most popular medical columnist in the United States. Dr. Gott lives with his wife and seven-year-old son in northwestern Connecticut, where he practices medicine and makes house calls.